AF873814

PALEO&PROTEIN

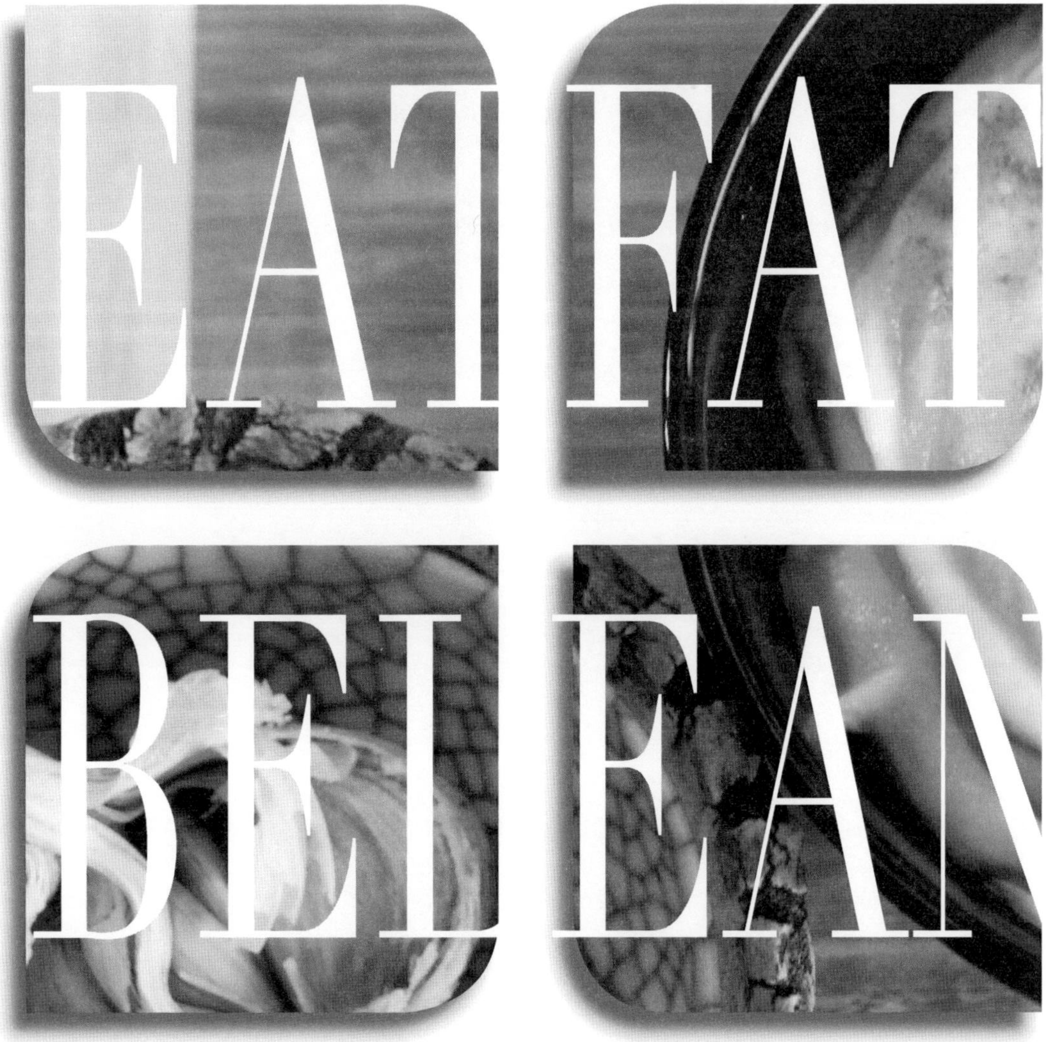

Andi Lew & Natalie Kringoudis

INSPIREDRECIPES

First published in Australia in 2013 by Heart to Heart Publishing
Address: 20 Ormond Rd Elwood VIC 3184
Tel: 0415-752311
Fax: 03-95313131
Email: andi_lew@yahoo.com
Website: www.eatfatbethin.com.au

Copyright © Andi Lew and Natalie Kringoudis 2013

All rights reserved. No part of this publication may be reproduced, stored in a retrieval system or transmitted in any form by any means, electronic, mechanical, photocopying, recording or otherwise, without the prior written permission of the publisher and copyright holder.

Andi Lew and Natalie Kringoudis assert the moral right to be identified as the authors of this work.

National Library of Australia Cataloguing-in-Publication entry

Author: Lew, Andi.
Title: Eat fat be Lean : Paleo and protein recipes / Andi Lew ; Natalie Kringoudis.
ISBN: 978-0-9873504-3-5 (Paperback)
ISBN: 978-0-9873504-1-1 (Ebook)
Subjects: Diet.
Cooking.
Other Authors/Contributors:
Kringoudis, Natalie.
Dewey Number: 613.25

www.eatfatbelean.com.au
www.andilew.com
www.thepagodatree.com.au

Cover photography by James Penlidis
Cover layout and design by Felicity Gilbert
Edited by Suzanne Male and Julie Postance
Printed by BPA printing

Typeset in Franklin Gothic Book 11pt on 15pt

Disclaimer

All care has been taken in the preparation of the information herein, but no responsibility can be accepted by the publisher or author for any damages resulting from the misinterpretation of this work. All contact details given in this book were current at the time of publication, but are subject to change.

The information in this book is provided for health education purposes and is not intended as medical advice. If you have any medical problems, please consult with a health care professional. The author and publisher shall not be responsible for any person with regard to any loss or damage caused directly or indirectly by the information in this book.

ABOUT THE AUTHORS

andi lew

A natural nurturer and advocate for healthy living, Andi Lew is a health professional, television presenter and author.

Andi is a qualified paediatric massage instructor, chiropractic assistant and a regular guest on radio and TV shows where she is often approached for advice on natural health and how to stay thin and fit.

She is a TV and radio personality presenting on a variety of shows about natural health and parenting. She writes regularly on health for magazines such as Ultra Fit and Australian Natural Health, and blogs for model mum Miranda Kerr's KORA Organics website.

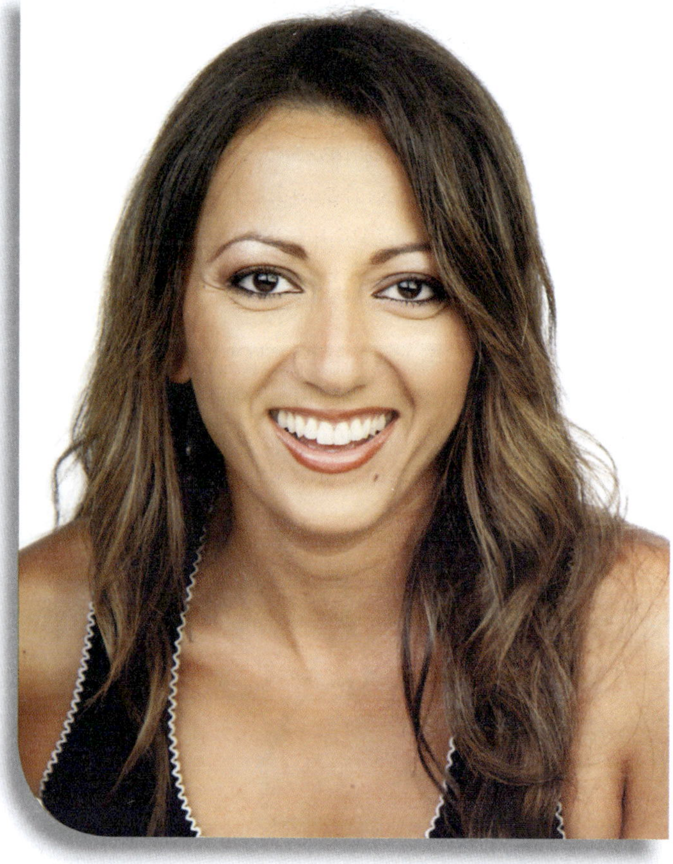

Andi is co-author of international top seller *7 Things Your Doctor Forgot to Tell You*, *Eat Fat Be Thin* and author of natural parenting guide *The Modern Day Mother*.

A dedicated mother and educator, you can visit her websites at www.andilew.com, www.themoderndaymother.com, www.eaftfatbethin.com.au and www.7things.com.au

ABOUT THE AUTHORS

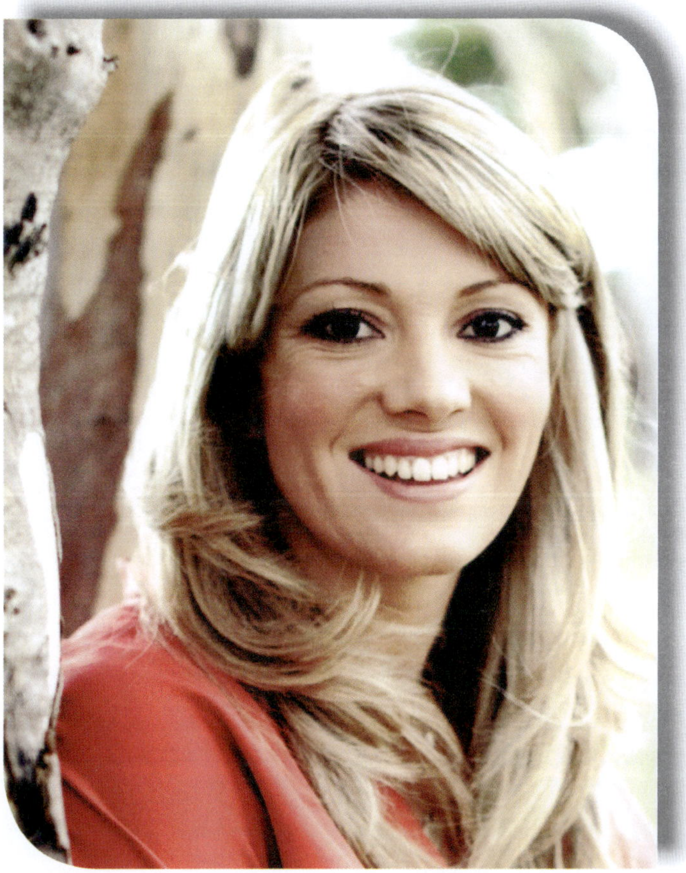

Natalie Kringoudis is a Doctor of Chinese Medicine, acupuncturist, natural fertility educator, speaker, author and producer. She is also the owner of The Pagoda Tree (www.thepagodatree.com.au), a hub for natural fertility and women's health in Australia.

Nat is on a crusade to share her knowledge to women and to open their hearts to the possibilities that arrive when they take control of their health and fertility.

She shares via her website www.melbournenaturalfertility.com.au and through her books and videos, reaching out to thousands of women in her quest to equip them with an abundance of information that will allow them to make their own well-informed health decisions.

Nat's dream is for all young women to understand how important their fertility is, knowing that fertility is simply having a healthy reproductive system, not necessarily about having a baby. She has recently gone on to produce & co-host her own web series, healthtalks. She is also the author of *Fertilise Yourself* and the co-author of *Eat Fat, Be Thin*.

natalie kringoudis

This is our second book
of its kind and we are back
by popular demand!

Our first book, **Eat Fat Be Thin** was launched in December 2012 and is jam packed with fantastic information, with lots of sweet treats full of good fats that help you lose weight.

Within a month, we sold out and went on to a second print run. We had feedback such as, "You had me at 'eat fat'."

Other feedback from our fans and followers were things like. "We want more recipes!" and "Can you do another book with savoury recipes?"

So, here we are! We have been working hard and brought you everything you need to keep you thin and lean!

thank you

A big thank you to Anthony and Jacob from J'Aton Couture for the fabulous dresses used on the cover, 2XU athletic wear, James Penlidis for the photography, Luke Perger for hair styling from Bouquet & Garter, Ellie Make-up *www.elliemakeup.com,* Gui Di Nardo, our sports model on the cover and to our friends and family for helping us bake, eat and photograph.

To our readers, thank you for purchasing this book. We had fun in the kitchen and hope you do too!

TABLE OF CONTENTS

TABLE OF CONTENTS

foreword

Having got the skinny on fat in their first book, Eat Fat Be Thin, you now get the whole deal with more recipes, greater insights and a better understanding on how and why fat not only tastes great but is actually good for you.

Over the last two decades, science has continued to reveal the benefits of good fats and oils and has repeatedly told us of the dangers of bad fat, but for some reason all we ever hear is the BAD STUFF! Well thankfully, once again, Andi and Nat have put together a healthy guide to eating fat and staying healthy and lean, that even includes recipes!

Having been in the health and wellness industry for nearly 20 years, I have seen a heap of trends and fads come and go. I've seen people be vegetarian (I've even been vegetarian), I've seen people only eat meat and animal fat (I've actually done Atkins!), and I've witnessed people avoid fat so much to the point where the only thing they eat is starchy carbs (fortunately I have never done that).

During this time the most depressing thing has been the massive rise in heart disease and cancer across the Western world. People are more depressed and stressed than ever before and in times like these, eating fat and protein can actually help us curb carb cravings as well as lift our mood and energy levels.

I've known Andi for years and it's rare to meet someone with so much unwavering passion for what she believes in. Despite the many detractors of health and wellbeing in the media, Andi continues to rise above the rubble of poor quality information and sheds bright new light on tricky subjects regarding health and individual health choices.

This healthy choice, eating fat, is particularly close to my heart and yours too. The fact is, if you think fat is bad, eat low fat as a rule and eat more carbs because you are scared of fat, you should be more scared now than ever before, because eating less fat and more carbs actually does increase your risk of heart disease and high cholesterol.

Teaming up with the awesome Dr Natalie Kringoudis brings a welcomed clash of philosophies, where East meets West, and Nat brings to the table eastern practice and philosophies on health and wellbeing. In yet again another win for the planet – Nat and Andi tackle the tricky subject surrounding our evolutionary predetermination and genetic coding, that if you take too seriously could do your head in. Nat and Andi have digested the relevant information about Paleo and have crafted an easy to follow, colloquial take on a Paleo/ Primal approach to living (eating well).

In reading this book you should feel a significant load of stress lifted from your shoulders from the guilt associated with eating fat. Having a better understanding of the relevance of protein, fat and carbohydrate in your diet is empowering, liberating and exciting. Because now, more than ever, eating fat isn't only good for you, it's TRENDY!

Well done Nat and Andi on this easy-to-read, bite-sized chunk of great information. It's a healthy, insightful and entertaining read that anyone can understand and enjoy straight away.

Dr Damian Kristof
B.Chiro N.D.

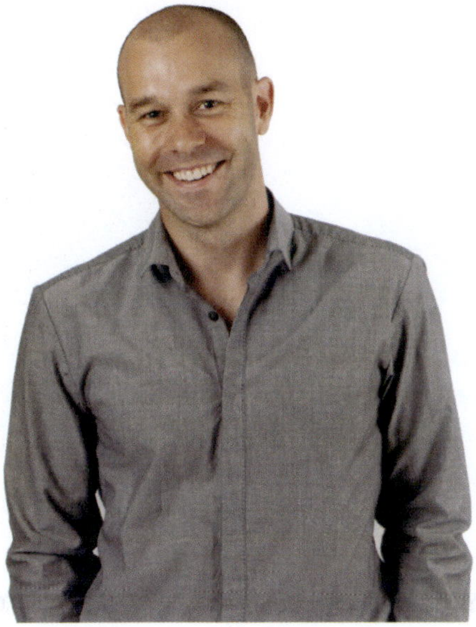

introduction

The big question is how do you eat fat and stay lean?

You'll soon learn by reading this book, not only will you become lean, but by eating this way, you will actually stay lean!

In the past we have trusted experts who have fed us advice on the dirty D-word: diet. And we believe food packaging that eating the low fat, low calorie products within will deliver weight loss.

In fact, since the 1980s, we've been told that reducing the amount of fat we eat is the key to losing weight, managing cholesterol and preventing health problems. But when it comes to your mental wellbeing and physical health, cutting the fat isn't the answer.

When the 'low fat' message hit our shores, cake was the first thing to go. But you are about to discover that the true secret of svelte doesn't require you to banish cake. You can have healthy sweet treats and foods filled with protein for muscle building.

The truth is we must include fat in our daily diet to stay thin – this is the secret to becoming lean!

Once you've digested that concept, sink your teeth into the reality of how much cake you've been missing out on and how much protein and vegetables you really should be eating too!

ok

so just how did we get so fat?

Good question! For years, many of us have done what we thought to be the right thing when it came to a healthy diet. But if it was so right, why did we continue to get fatter and fatter?

After being brainwashed into believing that fat is the

enemy, the idea of eating it seems crazy, and for many, really scary. Indeed, nothing changes the fact that fat is fat, but what we need to change is the notion that fat makes us fat.

You might be wondering where the fat actually comes from, especially the stuff that sits on your hips, butt and thighs, and gives you bingo wings or hail damage and cottage cheese buttocks!

Fat is actually your body's way of protecting itself. Fat literally grabs and traps toxins and tucks them out of harm's way to prevent poisonous matter from scooting around your blood stream and making you really sick. The thing is, over time, this causes huge health issues and at some point, your body begins to pack it in.

We love eating. We love baking and entertaining, but most of all, we just love eating tasty food.

Let's face it, who doesn't?

Before we found out the truth, we also wanted to have our cake and eat it too. We thought eating well was going to be boring, bland or time consuming. But we were wrong. We discovered a whole new world and began experimenting with easy and quick recipes that used fats our bodies love.

Being fat isn't necessarily a result of eating fat. It's a product of a toxic diet of highly processed, refined and sugary foods. Don't be fooled though: many fatty foods tick all the toxic boxes. We need to get back to wholesome living rather than 'hole-some' eating. We need to choose whole foods rather than foods that are empty in nutritional value, which contribute to this ever-growing weight problem.

We are so excited to share with you our favourite savoury treats. The good news is, not only are they delicious, but they are guilt free and darn good for your hips and your lips!

CHAPTERONE

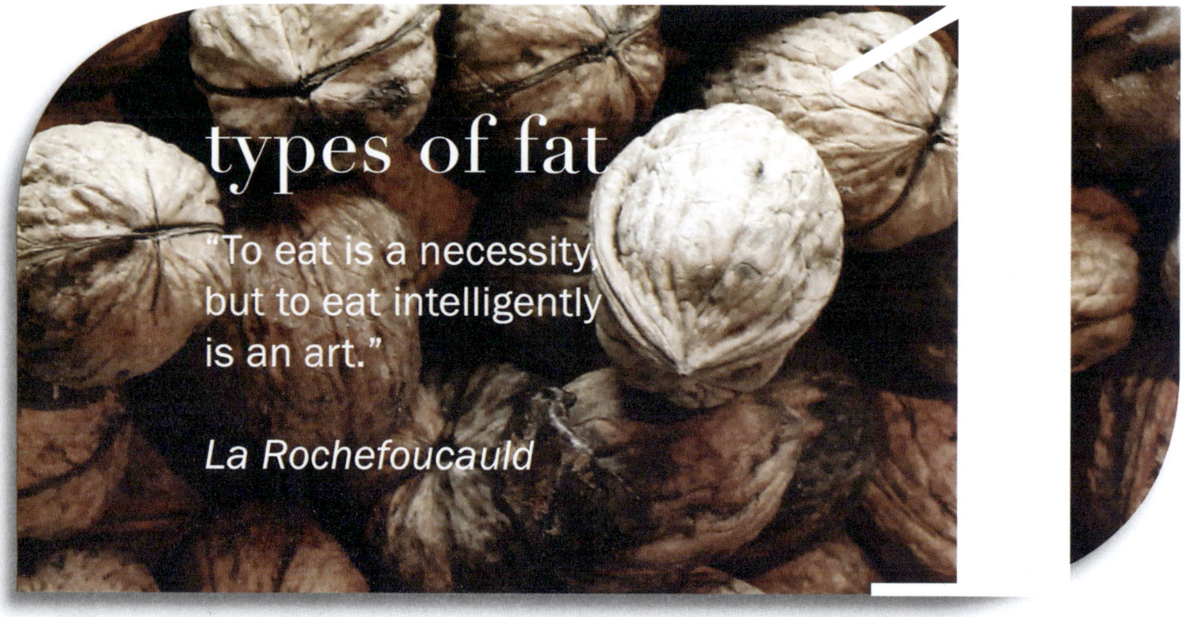

types of fat

"To eat is a necessity, but to eat intelligently is an art."

La Rochefoucauld

The type of fat you eat can mean the difference between fuel-up and blow-out. If you're into getting lean muscle, it may help you go from just fit to shredded.

'Eating clean' is a big term used by bodybuilders to describe foods that are fresh or without 'fat' or heavy sugary carbohydrates that are essential for your diet.

The Japanese diet has always been referred to as 'clean food'. Japanese people eat fresh, often raw fish and animal proteins and 'clean' vegetables - roots, greens and pickled varieties.

However, some weightlifters and 'gym junkies' may be stuck in the 'old school' modality, eating protein that may be older than their gym program, that usually comes from a tuna can, or simply avoiding 'fat' all together!

This chapter will reveal information about different types of fat that will empower you to make conscious, healthy living choices that will set you and your family up for long and happy lives, free from the burden of weight watching.

It will explain which proteins are best too, obviously, the fresher the better. The bonus is that when you learn about types of fats and how to use them, you achieve not only a better figure, but better health too.

Eating healthily no longer has to be boring. If you're going to eat, you may as well eat food that is guilt free and has maximum taste. The added bonus is that it is nutritious. And you're about to find out how eating our recommended fats and cakes, combined with a healthy, active lifestyle, can actually keep you lean.

Here's the 'low-down' on 'low fat'. The new 'black' is 'high fat'. You read it right! Low fat is a thing of the past. High fat is actually how we are designed to eat. Quality therapeutic fats will never make us fat. Our bodies do not store *good fat* as fat. You will soon discover how sugars do that and good fats help us to move fat.

There are four main types of fat - saturated, polyunsaturated, monounsaturated and trans fats. We need the first three in our diets because some fats are better for us than others. It's also important to become aware of the amounts of each of the fats you are eating. But ditch those trans fats!

Some fats are healthier to cook with than others. So let's look at each of the fats in turn.

fattype 1

SATURATEDFATS

Butter, lard, cream, other dairy, meat, poultry with skin on, cheese, fried foods.

Saturated fats include the foods above, which also contain dietary cholesterol. Many baked goods and fried foods can contain high levels of saturated fats. Some plant foods such as palm oil, palm kernel oil and coconut oil also contain primarily saturated fats, but do not contain cholesterol.

Saturated fats fall into two categories:

those that are high in saturated fatty acids (and therefore lower in unsaturated fatty acids), and those that are lower in saturated fatty acids (but higher in unsaturated fatty acids). The latter is much better for you and, as you will discover, many of our recipes contain plant foods that offer saturated fats, like coconut butter (or coconut oil – they are the same thing).

The benefits of the saturated fats from plants are vast; because of their therapeutic qualities they are key when it comes to eating fat and still being thin.

Coconut oil gets our seal of approval. It's just so versatile. Some oils become carcinogenic (cancer-causing) when heated at high temperatures, but not coconut oil. Look for cold-pressed organic coconut oil, which is exactly that – cold-pressed when it's extracted from the coconut. It's solidified, which means it makes a good butter alternative too.

Being able to cook with it at high temperatures is not the only great thing about coconut oil either. The properties in coconut oil are comparable to colostrum, since both coconut oil and mother's milk contain medium chain fatty acids that nourish, are easily absorbed and protect the body against illness.

The essential fatty acids are just that: essential. As part of healthy fats, they have a key role in maximising health. Consuming healthy fats, mean you can have fewer cravings and greater satisfaction because you feel fuller, and they help you burn more calories by increasing energy and metabolism – all this just by eating healthy fats! And here lies the big bonus: they may actually help you lose weight.

These reasons are why you'll see coconut oil in many of our recipes. In fact, using coconut in any form is extremely healthy for you. Try using shredded coconut. It's another 'super fat' and also super tasty in cakes and treats.

fattype2

POLYUNSATURATEDFATS

Vegetable oils, including soybean oil, corn oil and safflower oil, as well as fatty fish such as salmon, mackerel, herring and trout. Other sources include some nuts and seeds such as walnuts and sunflower seeds.

Omega 3 and omega 6 are found in many foods high in polyunsaturated fats (think oily fish, nuts and seeds) and are your friends for cardiovascular health. These are key fats to include in your diet and are especially vital for the expecting mother, who will need this type of nutrition for both her and her growing new baby. It's awesome brain food! Omega 3 fatty acids are essential for healthy foetal development, but are also wonderful for healthy skin, good vision and overall wellness, right down to treating mood disorders and moving post-baby weight.

As well as being an excellent way of getting essential fatty acids, nuts and seeds are also an excellent source of protein for vegans and vegetarians.

fattype3

MONOUNSATURATEDFATS

Vegetable oils such as olive oil, canola oil, peanut oil, sunflower oil and sesame oil. Other sources include avocados, peanut butter, and many nuts and seeds.

Related to these three main types of fat are trans fats. Trans fats are unsaturated fats (mostly from plants) that have been hydrogenated, which means they have had hydrogen added to them. This process usually happens in food processing, particularly in the production of hard margarines. In fact, margarine is so processed that it is actually black in colour when first produced then a yellow dye is added to it to make it look pretty. Scary?

Even more shocking news is that margarine is one molecule away from being plastic. Stick it outside in direct sunshine and it fails to melt. And we eat this? Worse still is the notion that eating specific margarines is the means to lower cholesterol.

We're not advocates of eating near plastic to lower cholesterol. There is increasing evidence that trans fats are probably the worst of all fats for our health.

But it's not all bad news when it comes to monosaturated fats. Avocados (which also contain polyunsaturated fat) are an amazing source of monosaturated fat and provide an outstanding nutritional advantage, especially when it comes to weight loss and hormone function.

Get avocados into your system any way you can: put them in salads or a salsa dip, on rye crackers with a slice of a favourite vegetable, or eat with a spoon and some cracked pepper and sea salt.

The best way to incorporate these types of fats into your daily diet is to eat nuts and seeds often. It's a myth to avoid eating too many nuts. Of course, we should have a varied diet but nuts and seeds should be a plenty, along with fresh vegetables.

Nuts are a part of the Paleo diet, which we will learn more about soon. They should still be eaten in moderation. One kind of fat, omega 6 is best eaten in smaller amounts although still essential. The other kind, omega 3 fats can be enjoyed a little more freely. They are high in mono-unsaturated fats and have been shown in numerous clinical trials to lower cholesterol.

So bring on the nuts! In the list below you'll see our best recommendations as to which nuts can be consumed in higher quantities due to their specific properties and which should be consumed less – this has to do with their omega ratios and nutrient content.

NUT/SEED

Almonds
Walnuts
Macadamia nuts
Pecans
Pine nuts

Cashews
Pistachio nuts
Hazelnuts
Chestnuts
Pumpkin seeds
Sunflower seeds

Try to buy raw and unsalted nuts. Nut pastes and organic varieties are popular too now. Loving Earth is a company that is dedicated to creating activated nuts so you can buy many great products through them but we will also show you how to make them in our recipes section.

Activated nuts do amazing things for your insides and are super easy to make yourself (not to mention much more cost effective). Why 'activate' them? Sounds like something cartoon characters do before they are about to jump off the roof of a burning building - "Activate systems - go!" Well, it's kind of like that - when you soak nuts, they sprout, activating all the goodness. By eating these as a snack, you're doing your digestion a big favour, promoting better absorption and increasing health. And remember, your gut is the pivot of your health and fertility. When it has everything it needs to fuel your body it all just works. These need to make their way into your pantry.

Listen to your body and see how including these good fats feel for you. Remember, while they are not meant to be a staple, they are certainly a crucial, or essential, part of our diets.

Avocados target the health and function of the womb and cervix of the female – they even look just like these organs, with the shape replicating the womb and the seed, the baby. When a woman eats one avocado a week, it balances hormones, sheds unwanted birth weight and helps prevent cervical cancers. And how profound is this fact? It takes exactly nine months to grow an avocado from blossom to ripened fruit.

(Excerpt taken from Natalie's book, Fertilise Yourself)

the magic of COCONUT OIL

Coconut oil is your best friend. It actually helps you lose weight, even more so than other fats. This is because it is composed of a very special and unique group of saturated fats known as medium-chain triglycerides.

These types of fats deliver a 'swag' of health benefits because they are easily broken down in the gut – our favourite is weight loss! This is because unlike other fats, they do not require digestive enzymes secreted by the pancreases or bile from the gall bladder for digestion, therefore they actually bypass a stage in assimilation.

Most fats are digested in the small intestine where bile and pancreatic digestive enzymes are secreted to break down the fatty acids. Ordinarily, these are absorbed into the intestinal wall, packaged into little sacs of fat and proteins known as lipoproteins and sent around the bloodstream. During circulation they release fat.

However, these medium chain triglycerides found in coconut oil are processed in a different manner, broken down into individual fatty acids before they leave the stomach. So when they arrive at the small intestine, they don't require any further attention, nor do they have the same effect as other fats do. This is why coconut oil assists in weight loss – this type of fat is readily used as fuel immediately.

We are huge fans of coconut oil – it is high in antimicrobial and antibiotic properties, it helps boost energy, increases metabolism and aids in keeping lean and shredding extra fat. There's nothing not to like about this little gem. Make it your BFF (best friend forever) too!

fat type 4

TRANSFATS

Trans fats can be found in many foods like margarine, but especially in fried foods like French fries and doughnuts, in baked goods including pastries, pie crusts, biscuits, pizza dough, cookies and crackers, and in stick margarines and shortenings.

You can determine the amount of trans fats in a particular packaged food by looking at the nutritional panel on the side of the package.

The most important thing to get from this section is DO NOT EAT trans fats. They have been chemically altered and because of this, offer very little nutritional benefit. Basically, anything that is too processed or altered from its natural state is not really 'food' anymore.

Try to eat things that are as close to nature as possible. Trans fats are much more harmful to body function than saturated fats, and therefore should be avoided.

However do not fret, because you can still have your cake and it eat it too! This book has a variety of tasty recipes that do not use any trans fats. You will not miss out and can still eat everything from torte to tart and cupcake to cake.

'Diet' food can taste great and doesn't have to be bland. Dinner parties will have your guests talking for days, not only about how delicious your food was, but also how it helped them stay lean too.

Next time you get invited to someone's house for dinner or tea and cake, you may like to bring your own 'healthy' version you learned to make from this book. Why not spread the love around? Or try making something that you can take to work for lunch, creates conversation with colleagues and lays on the lean talk!

Some of these oils do a have a place in your pantry. Olive, peanut, quality sunflower and sesame oil can be great for pouring, meaning they will not only make your salad or dish taste delicious, but will make it nutritious too. Canola oil is best avoided as it is genetically engineered and doesn't tick any 'health favour' boxes for this reason.

CHAPTER TWO

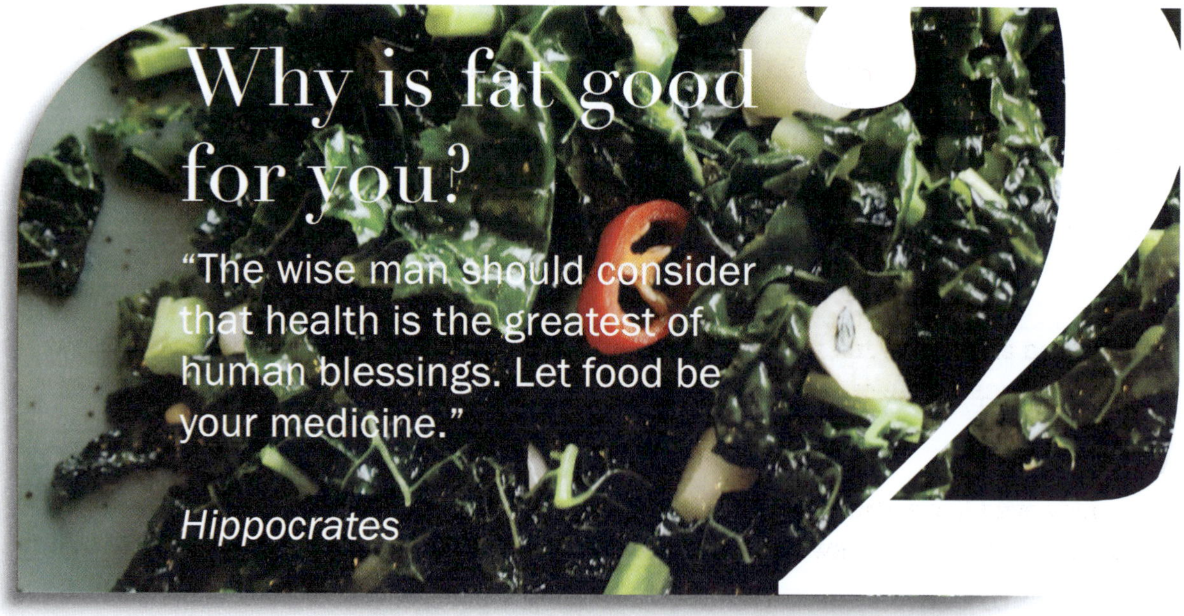

Why is fat good for you?

"The wise man should consider that health is the greatest of human blessings. Let food be your medicine."

Hippocrates

Fat has been the big, bad wolf when it comes to being and looking thin and fit. Health-conscious people across the globe are buying 'low fat', 'light' and fewer calorie options when it comes to food. "Oh, don't touch that cake!" and "A moment on the lips, a lifetime on the hips!" are phrases we have all heard before. However, somewhere along the line we have tipped the scales, grabbed the life jackets and headed for a sinking boat, despite our best efforts to stay thin and be healthy.

The truth is that fat is actually good for you. And that's not all. It also helps you lose weight when you eat the right types of fat.

The health benefits of eating the right fats are many. They are absolutely essential in a diet, hence the term Essential Fatty Acids (EFAs). Without them we would miss out on vital nutrients - vitamins A, D and E that are needed to prevent or control all kinds of symptoms and conditions such as heart disease, cancers, immune system deficiencies, arthritis, skin complaints, PMS and menopausal symptoms. They are also critical for nervous system function, brain development and for healthy reproductive function, as hormones are made of fats and proteins.

Is it any wonder then why we are seeing women's health problems on the rise at the same time women's hips are growing? The scales have been tipped way too far in the wrong direction.

Low fat foods have been linked to infertility in both men and women. As we discussed earlier, this is because they don't contain the adequate nutrients that their full-fat siblings provide. Whole foods are always, hands down, the best option. And there are extra benefits. You can end up with a stronger immune system or become more fertile.

Fats are also a great source of energy and because they don't store water, they can be used to store almost twice the amount of energy compared to protein or carbohydrate.

Fats have huge benefits. So there's nothing to be afraid of, or send you running to the treadmill. Take a deep yoga breath and relax knowing that the best news of all is: fats make us full; they help us to feel satiated so we don't overeat. Genius!

SO when did we get so scared of fat?

In a nutshell, fat was blamed for heart disease. American scientist Ancel Keys observed that people who had a diet high in fat were more likely to develop heart disease, so he went on a crusade encouraging people to cut the fat. His logic was that when you ate fat, this same fat transferred to your heart, arteries and around your organs.

But most of the cultures he observed had the same Western way of eating. Had he gathered information using several more cultural groups like the Greeks or Inuits, he would have found that some cultures have a diet high in fat yet have low rates of heart disease.

We also need to learn that cholesterol is actually good. We can help ourselves by eating good cholesterol. And you thought that we had to steer clear of it because it was a no-no?

You'll be pleased to know that:

- our hormones are made of cholesterol – especially our sex hormones.
- the fat we have circulating in our system is saturated (saturated or monounsaturated fat) since we are essentially animals and this is a vital life ingredient that we make ourselves or get from our food (but not necessarily from saturated fat).
- eggs are good fats. But know this: free-range eggs/organic eggs contain 50% more omega oils than battery range eggs.

Throw away the old notion that too many eggs are bad for you. Since we can regularly eat eggs, it seems there isn't necessarily 'good' and 'bad' cholesterol, but rather just cholesterol.

To cut a long story short, the types of food we eat will contribute to the levels of cholesterol present in the body. The higher amount of cholesterol present, the more danger it poses to your health. But remember, we do need some cholesterol in our bodies – at least enough to produce our hormones.

Saturated and trans fats influence cholesterol the most. What research has now found is that a diet low in fat can potentially shoot your cholesterol levels through the roof. On top of this, most low fat foods you encounter are full of fructose, which is the type of sugar that makes us fat. So the combination of a food being low fat and also lacking nutritional value is disastrous.

So how much fat can you have? Good question. This is tricky to answer since we aren't all built the same. Most of the recipes you will find in this book combine fat and protein, which is a darn good mix, not just for your taste buds; it also makes your health go gangbusters.

So, does this mean we should eat less saturated fat since it increases cholesterol? That really depends on what you replace it with. You now know that if you were to replace saturated fat with low fat options or hydrogenated products you'd be gearing to jump up a few dress sizes and cause some terrible strain on your innards. But if you replaced the saturated fats with polyunsaturated fats, you'd be doing yourself, your heart and your buttocks a favour!

The thing is, the body can't make monounsaturated and polyunsaturated fats. It must get them from dietary sources, so it is essential to pump up the intake to move toward better health. The best combo is less saturated fats and more of the polyunsaturated and monounsaturated varieties.

So there is nothing wrong with eating an egg a day. In fact, you could have seven. They are a perfect food and provide all the nutrients we need. You could probably survive on a diet of eggs. Many of our cakes in our first book, Eat Fat, Be Thin use eggs, so hooray for our hormones, health and happiness!

CHAPTER THREE

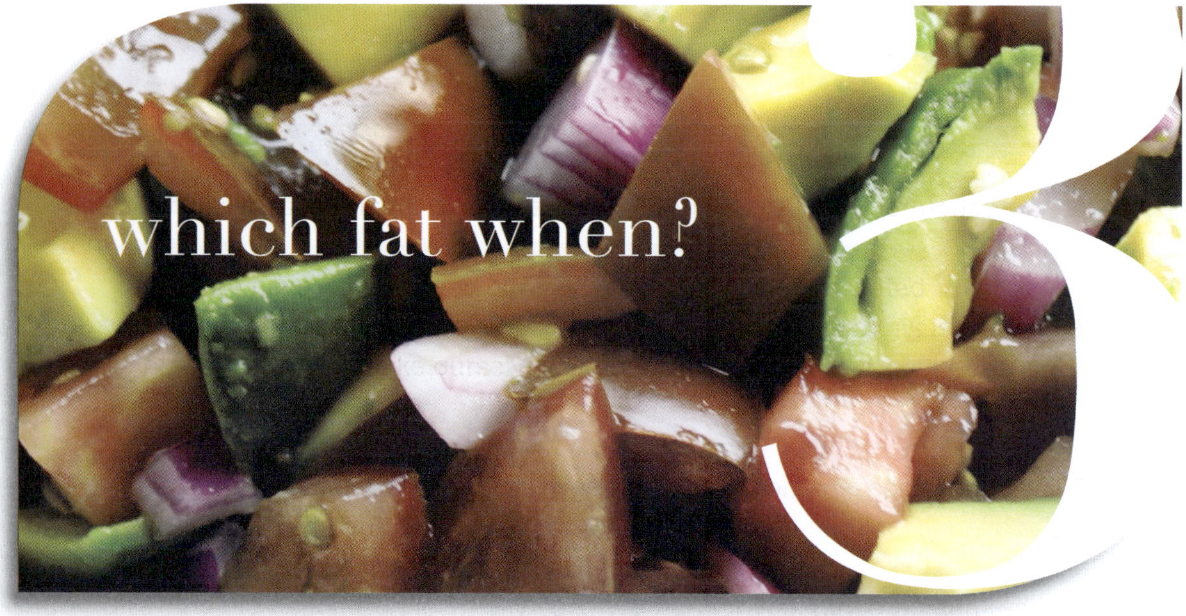

which fat when?

SO

how much of the good stuff can we have?

As a general rule, to maintain great health and good nutrition, we need a rough mix of all three:

1. **protein**
2. **low GI carbohydrates, and**
3. **therapeutic fats.**

Roughly 20-30% of this should be made up of these therapeutic fats.

However, the mix of fats that you eat, rather than the total amount in your diet, is what matters most when it comes to your cholesterol and health. The key is to eat more good fats and less bad fats. Isn't it great that we are now including cholesterol in this list?

So, a perfect example of a daily intake of fats may be:

BREAKFAST

Eggs
Eat them whatever way you like them. They are a complete meal. We like to fry them with coconut butter.

SNACK

Nuts and seeds, vegetable sticks, snow peas, steamed broccoli or baked sweet potato.

LUNCH

Corn taco shell with black beans or chicken, salsa and avocado. Use chia seed oil.

SNACK

Veggie sticks with hommus or a coconut milk smoothie with coconut oil or coconut yoghurt.

DINNER

Salmon steak and salad with good cold-pressed organic oil.

See a more complete food plan, as well as a shopping directory in Chapter 6.

a clever diet

The best way to fuel your body is to eat foods that are as close to nature as possible. The more alive your foods are, the more life they will have and therefore give you. So make fresh fruits and vegetables your main source and include protein in every meal. Muscles need protein to grow and women in general don't eat enough. It does not need to be meat. You can get protein sources from boiled eggs, nuts (which contain fats – extra bonus!), goat's cheese, quinoa and lean meats.

Eating fats in all meals means knowing which are good to eat, and which you need to ditch.

EATUP

With saturated fats, good fats for hot uses are coconut and palm oils, biodynamic butter, eggs, meat and seafood. Good unsaturated fats for cold uses are olive oil, sesame, nut, flaxseed, avocado and chia seed oils.

ditch saturated fats like margarine, hydrogenated oils or even partly hydrogenated oils and oil-blend margarines. Say bye-bye to these unsaturated bad guys too:

canola, corn, vegetable, soybean, grapeseed, sunflower, safflower and rice bran oils. They're all highly processed.

Add that to the fact that you could get some of that intake by eating from one of our recipes and you will think this new diet is literally a 'piece of cake'.

Notice something is missing? Yes, that's flour and bread. The ingredients we use in the recipes do not contain wheat. We prefer to use flours that don't contain gluten, including coconut flour, rice flour, millet flour and sometimes spelt flour.

Spelt contains gluten but is a very easily digested grain and doesn't upset the stomach unlike its sibling, whole-wheat flour. If you are gluten intolerant, recipes like our Orange and Chia Seed Cake in our book, Eat Fat, Be Thin are perfect for you. The almond meal and coconut flours are gluten free, very nutritious and high in essential fatty acids and protein.

The Aussie brand, Forage, has a great range of cereals too that are wheat and gluten free and they taste delicious.

Wheat contains gluten, which is a protein that is really difficult to digest and has been linked with a host of health problems including depression, migraines and cancer among others.

When we eat it, our gut goes into inflammation frenzy as it tries to digest it, and over time our adrenals become exhausted with this constant reaction to the inflammation in the intestines. The result can be a very sick, tired and fat body.

Yes, wheat can make you fat because it is converted to sugar and also because eventually the adrenals have no capacity left to produce the necessary hormones to digest. Perhaps this reaction may not have been as bad had we not genetically modified wheat so that it grew better, faster and was more resilient to bugs and droughts.

As you can see, there's no end to eating fat. It's the wheat and sugar-converted fat that sits on your body that is the enemy. We learn about the other 'food' that is fat disguised as sugar in the next chapter. The real fat oils slide through your system, making your body run like a well-oiled engine. Go enjoy it all day and every day as long as it's the right stuff.

PHATEXERCISE

We're all guilty of doing it. Before we knew any better, we exercised like fools with countless hours of running on the treadmill and the same workout regime, week after week. The most ironic part of the story is that there were little results. We still struggled to keep the weight off because we were misinformed and on the low fat bandwagon.

The combination of a low fat, low-nutrient and boring exercise regime was achieving terrible results. But we kept on going because what other option did we have? What a breath of fresh air it is to grasp the concept of eating for wellness and health: eating fat and exercising right. Who knew it could be this easy?

It wasn't much fun, that daily 60-minute run on the tready, where living on the edge and 'pumping up the volume' meant sprinting every minute or so. Good riddance to boring workouts. In fact, high-level cardio is actually counter-productive because our bodies aren't made to work out that way. Not only that, it's a sure fire way to lose muscle mass if you are participating in too much cardiovascular exercise.

But back up the buggy there. Before you run for the hills, you must know that exercise is good. Very good. You need it. We all need it, but exercising right is key – and not exercising with the main focus being to lose weight.

Exercising to be healthy is right on the money. Exercise is vital for every part of us – the physical and the mental – as it aids in hormone regulation. It's the best way to move cortisol (the stress hormone) out of your body, and better still, the endorphins that are released after a workout are equally as good as the recipes in this book.

Varied exercise is the best form of exercise. In fact, it is how our bodies are designed to work out because it uses all muscle groups consistently. So sports like martial arts or gymnastics are good examples, as opposed to isolating muscle groups with weight programmes, which are useless. When you activate your core and engage all muscle groups, you will aid metabolism, which is fuelled by ... fats.

Personal trainers are now incorporating activities like 'strong man training' into their workouts whereby pulling, pushing and lifting things are all part of the regime. Here, most muscles groups are all activated at one time. So by eating fat, you are providing your body with the right energy it needs to perform these tasks, and because it is using it as energy, you are burning it. Another genius moment.

EXERCISEIDEAS

- CrossFit
- Jiu Jitsu
- Gymnastics
- Surfing
- Hiking
- Iyengar Yoga
- Boot camps
- Strong Man competitions (pulling, lifting and pushing exercises)
- Abseiling
- Kite surfing
- Iron Man competitions
- Triathlons
- Kayaking
- White water rafting
- Rock climbing – indoor or outdoor

There are many different exercise groups that offer this. Think outdoorsy, nature types of exercise. Variety is essential to keep you interested and your body guessing. Getting in the garden and landscaping, cutting down trees, lugging logs, carting full wheelbarrows or picking up sandbags and plants are all excellent types of exercise.

The way in which you pick up heavy things is important too. You only have to have a conversation with your doctor or chiropractor to know the importance of this, but from a perspective of how we are designed, we are meant to squat. And when we lift heavy things, we must 'bend our knees' they say, but what they mean is 'shut up and squat!'

It doesn't mean you shouldn't go for a walk around the block or a jog if you feel like it from time to time. Movement is exactly what your body needs. Being fit is one part of being healthy, just as eating fat is another. So the exercise you choose is just as important as the fat you choose. How much should you exercise? The answer is just as often as you eat good fat: often.

You need to aim to move your body several times daily. You'll also need to challenge your body with cardiovascular exercise a few times a week. If you sit at a computer all day, get up at least once an hour and walk around and do something that moves your body for five minutes.

This is especially essential for those who work long hours or those in high-pressure roles who experience periods of varying stress. When we are stressed, the hormone cortisol builds up in our systems. Movement is our body's natural way of moving this out. If cortisol builds up, it becomes toxin within us and can cause a host of issues including fertility troubles and weight gain.

During the work day it doesn't necessarily mean you need to get up and sprint every hour. This type of movement could be stretching gently or taking the garbage outside or hanging some washing.

Your activities need to be enjoyed at least a few times a week, so this may mean a hike, a surf and a gym class in a week, or three sessions of Brazilian Jiu-Jitsu, or gymnastics twice a week and a walk with hill sprints to make up another day.

Make sure you choose something that you find enjoyable so you look forward to going. It may be something you've never tried before or it may also mean needing to bring the kids with you. If you have little ones, you may like to wear your baby or toddler. The best baby carrier around is the Ergo Carrier, which is best for both the wearer and the child. The benefits of baby wearing are abundant but one of the benefits is that it helps the parent get fit.

On the days you are having 'off' from your activities and exercise routine, be sure to go for a gentle walk for 30 minutes to an hour. This could be incidental exercise where you choose to walk the neighbour's dog or perhaps walk to work instead of driving one day.

Once you make movement part of your lifestyle, you will have more energy as you release these hormones. This will also give your mental wellbeing a healthy boost. Then, right after your sessions, be sure to enjoy your good fats! Fill up on some quality fat like a handful of macadamia nuts and you are most certainly on the right track.

CHAPTER FOUR

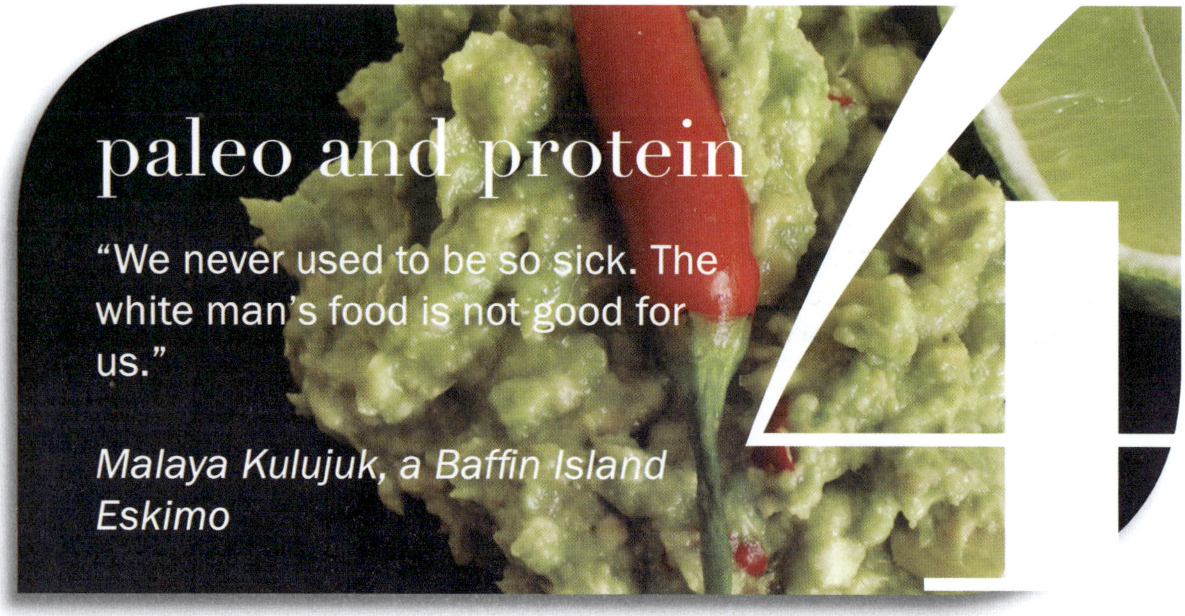

4 paleo and protein

"We never used to be so sick. The white man's food is not good for us."

Malaya Kulujuk, a Baffin Island Eskimo

The way we live today is very different to how we used to, or how we are designed to live. Many of the chronic illnesses of the Western world are a product of our lifestyle and what we now eat or don't eat.

We are primal creatures, born with three parts to our brain: mammalian, reptilian and primal brains, that then integrate to become one brain when we reach the age of about five to seven.

As primal creatures, our needs are simple and we are designed to breastfeed as infants, then slowly introduce foods that are picked, plucked, hunted or gathered.

This is natural. We were not meant to fill bellies with white breads and donuts, grains that are processed and bloat out on wheat cereals.

However, even though we have evolved as a species, the way our brains are designed have not. So one thing that sticks and does not change in our infant years, is the need for breast milk and natural whole foods that are as close to nature as possible.

The Paleo diet is actually ancient. '**Paleo**' is short for '**Paleolithic**', a term that refers to an era between 2 million and 10,000 years BC. It often relates to the lifestyle lived during the time of 'cavemen and women' as well as the 'hunter/gatherer' era. During this period, the way in which we lived was about foods that we once again could pick, pluck, hunt and gather.

The primal way of living is a great foundation to still go from after these infant years. This is what we will focus on, using Paleo as a guide for our modern world diet.

The Palaeolithic lifestyle lays a great foundation. That said, we like to focus on intuitive eating or primal eating and appreciate what works for one individual may not work for the next. Getting to understand what your own body requires is key to setting up healthy eating habits. The key is always whole foods; non-processed food which is as close to nature as possible.

however,

times haven't changed too much at all. You are the same as you have always been. Genetically speaking, we are virtually identical to our ancestors living over forty thousand years ago. To be here today, we have had to hunt, gather, pick and pluck our food, live through ice ages, scavenge and learn to survive in the environment around us.

But let's drill down. Physiologically you are the same as your forefathers living in the Paleolithic Era, far before tractors, chook pens and wheat silos. Your physiological make up is the same as the people from Paleolithic times.

In fact, for the entire stretch of human existence, we have been hunters. The huge difference is, what they were hunting hundreds of thousands of years ago was indeed chemical-free, absolutely free range and definitely not grain fed.

These ancestors ate large volumes of high quality animal source protein. With this, they consumed a decent amount of fat too – including saturated, monounsaturated and our personal favourites, omega 3s and 6s. After the Ice Age, a variety of vegetable matter was added to the diet including seeds, nuts and berries when in season.

While our genes are old, our modern diets are not. Our new food revolution, it seems, has only been around a very short time with packaged this and that, and low fat options. Considering how long humans have been roaming the earth, it makes sense for us to ditch the new diets and move to embrace the 'old' again.

So here's what we have taken from the 'old' and would like you to put in your 'new' primal or Paleo inspired diet:

- Good fats for example were very prominent in the primal living way of life as they were picked and plucked and a food that was crucial in a paleo diet. In our modern days, it is one thing that we forgot to include in our diet as we have been brainwashed into thinking fat was bad.

But good fat can help prevent cardiovascular disease. They are what your health practitioners would call 'cardio-protective' because they protect the heart and blood vessels from disease.

- An overload of acidic foods, which are packaged and cereal based, cheese filled, salty and fried foods with added excessive sodium (salt) generate an acidic overload in the body. This causes numerous health problems, particularly as we age and the body becomes less adaptable to handling the acid load.

  In previous times, we ate alkalizing foods like fresh fruits and vegetables, which buffered the acid from meat rich diets - this lifestyle is known as 'Paleo'. This is another crucial food group, dark greens which are alkaline and serve to balance the body back to health if you are including meat in your diet.

- Even though animal protein has been an important part of our diets over the years and we are designed to eat meat, just how much is the question. Some people's systems go gangbusters when increasing the quantity of meat consumed and others, not so much.

  Vegans and vegetarians who prefer to live a Vego-Paleo inspired life eating large amounts of nuts and seeds for protein need to be mindful just how vital protein is a key ingredient of our diet. The amino acids found in meat are essential to balancing hormones. These are not found in any other sources of food.

  It isn't as simple as cutting out meat without serious consideration of supplementation through other elements in your diet. You may need to further investigate what works best for you. The way we see it, meat wasn't always readily available on the table every minute of the day in Paleolithic times.

  Small animals were hunted and large animals may have been stumbled upon from time to time. This meant that we feasted on it when it was available and relied on other sources of nutrients when it wasn't at hand.

As we've evolved, foods have become readily available and convenient to source – but remember, quality meats – grass fed, grass finished is key. It isn't necessarily about quantity here.

You see, scientific evidence tells us over and over again that if our ancestors didn't eat meat, we wouldn't be here – in fact, we'd be more like our closest animal relative, the chimpanzee!

Chimps live mostly on a plant-based diet with a few eggs and insects thrown in for good measure. They sport the spare tyre, a big belly that is characteristic of vegetarian animals. For these animals to be able to digest, break down and assimilate the nutrients from all their fibrous plant food, their bellies must accommodate.

Thankfully we've evolved – we're no longer hairy and we don't have big guts! Not that there's anything wrong with that! Right? (winks!)

convert

STRICTPALEOFORPALEO-INSPIRED ANDPRIMALEATING

Our Paleo ancestors got clever (we're talking over 2.5 million years ago) and swapped their big bellies for larger brains, all because they worked out intuitively that eating animal proteins and fats gave them more stamina. That energy that was once needed to digest all the plant fibre was no longer required and as a result, the size of their brains began to grow and their tummies shrunk.

Studies of ancient and fossilized human faeces revealed very little or no evidence of plant material. These ancestors of ours survived primarily on fat – from animals. It was the key element of their diet for nutrients and energy. It was mostly marrow fat that provided them with nourishment, which also helped their guts to shrink and resulted in scavenged brains which contained docosahexaenoic acid or DHA that helped their brains to grow.

swap

SOMEMEAT FORMOREFAT!

DHA is essential for brain development. In fact, the latest research shows that children who are fed DHAs (think offal, organ meats and fish) are said to be up to five times more intelligent than children who don't.

As time went on, the climate warmed to reveal root vegetables, berries and seeds and they were able to add these fibrous plants to the diet but only as they were in season.

As you and I know, the climate was temperamental and often the environment meant the land was flooded or barren for long periods of time. Still they survived on the land, hunting and gathering what they could in their surroundings.

But, they survived because of fat. Not because they were fat, but because fat is our most efficient, dense and prolonged-burning fuel. It is one of the key elements to survival – and since you are a carbon copy of your ancestors, we all still require this same fat in our diet today.

Excerpt from Fertilise Yourself

I suspect that our forefathers (and mothers!) knew a whole lot more about nutrition intuitively than we give them credit for. Sure, they didn't have labs to nut down exactly what foods contained, better still it seems, they had a sound knowledge of food for medicine. They ate to

fuel the **body,**

to nourish & to heal

They realised, by observation, that some foods worked really well together and others were a fizzle. They weren't necessarily brain surgeons – but they listened to their bodies and their brains told them how to eat and why.

They observed the changes that food made and they were ever so clever to just 'know.' Why? Because they had time. Time to stop and observe. On top of that, food didn't come wrapped in plastic. It was eaten exactly as intended – whole. No skim milk or low fat mayo, and they weren't fat! They ate to live and in turn, they were a whole lot more fertile than we are today.

You see, eating for fertility isn't rocket science. All it involves is a heap of common sense. Clinically I don't apply a one-size-fits-all approach when it comes to treatment. BUT we do know that eating a certain way will undoubtedly benefit your fertility. This is the same for everybody as we were designed to eat for health.

Now we know that essential vitamins and minerals found in plants, seeds and nuts help make up a well balanced Paleolithic diet – however this wasn't always the case.

You see, prior to genetically modified foods, plants required cooking to remove toxins. Prior to the discovery of fire, these foods were either not available (during the Ice Age) or avoided because they were known to be indigestible. Once our ancestors could prepare their food over fire, they learnt to cook out these toxins.

Today, we have genetically modified many of the poisonous plant foods to remove the toxins. The problem with this is that our bodies just aren't designed to eat such foods raw anyway – remember, we have those same genetics!

In fact, for many of us, eating a large volume of raw foods can cause a host of gut-related issues and lead to weight gain. This is because our bodies digest food at 37 °C.

Overconsumption of raw and uncooked foods not only forces the gut to work some serious overtime to digest, but it also first has to raise the temperature of the food before it can effectively deal with it.

We hope by now you may have some type of understanding of what works for your body and why. Maybe you already know that you can't tolerate gluten (most of us can't) or that beans send you running to the bathroom!

You've learnt that through tuning into your body and listening, you know what works and what doesn't. We know you're interested in becoming a better version of yourself. You have this book in your hands teaching you things you intuitively know. The rat race surely has disconnected us from our ability to tune in. We're just here to remind you.

How much protein please?

The exact amount of protein we require will differ from person to person – we are all unique individuals; we have different genetics, environments and constitutions. That said, if we are the same as we have always been, the requirements of just how much protein we require falls within a range and hasn't changed in the last several thousand years (if ever).

The approximate recommended dietary intake for most adults is between 45-55 grams each meal. The best way to consume this is to break it up throughout the day so that every meal and snack you consume has some element of protein in it.

Since we encourage you to avoid grains, breads, pasta and sugars it becomes easier to get your head around exactly where your protein is coming from. The best sources of protein are high-quality, nutrient-rich and complete. Our bodies require these for repair, regeneration and rebuilding of muscle and tissues. These might look like wild caught salmon, grass fed and grass finished meats and organic, free range eggs.

According to Nora Gedgaudas (Author of *Primal Body, Primal Mind*), the method to calculate the exact (or nearest to) amount of protein each individual requires is 0.08g per kilo of body weight. That said, some with very poor digestive systems may require up to 10g or more.

Body builders and athletes require more – up to 1.5g of actual protein per kilo of body weight. A typical body builder's intake may be 150g of protein, six times a day. It is always best to consult with your trainer and health professional and keep monitoring how your body is responding.

You may have heard that high protein diets get a bad rap. This is mostly because people seek out poor quality foods and proteins, which can lead to ill health. It's so important to consider how digestible the food is, how close to nature it is, as well as the ability of your digestive system to assimilate your meals. We'll talk about the importance of a healthy digestive system soon.

Too much protein may lead to too much pooping!

As we've established, we can only tolerate a certain amount of protein – around 200-300 grams per day depending on how many kilos you're pushing. Too much protein will see you running to the bathroom, can cause nausea or send you to an early grave if the balance isn't right.

Our Paleolithic ancestors realised we couldn't simply live on lean muscle meat alone. Adding fat to the mix was and still is the perfect combination. Plant proteins that provide carbohydrates are also valuable – but the real deal for us is the fat and protein balance. Too much lean protein has toxic effects. The solution –

fat!

Large animals have a higher fat to protein ratio. Think cow and deer, which contain more fat and less protein. Smaller animals like chickens and rabbits have a lesser amount of fat – the squirrel's body is 83 per cent protein and 17 per cent fat. The mule deer's body is 40 per cent protein and 60 per cent fat.

If the only protein on your plate was squirrel for several months, you would rapidly head toward protein toxicity. The fat and lean meat combination is crucial for wellness which is why our Paleolithic grandfathers risked their lives to seek out larger animals. They were well aware of protein toxicity.

With your Paleolithic lifestyle, you are well cared for and not at risk of protein toxicity as we encourage quality produce added to each meal. And because our friend, the omega 3s are in good quantities in our diets, as well as alkalising greens, we are well protected from heart disease or cholesterol issues.

Your best protein options

You don't necessarily have to kit up in your Paleolithic Flintstone flavoured fashion and go hunting in order to live your new Primal lifestyle! The staple foods to set you up are available at your local market or supermarket.

These include meats (including organ meats), fish and seafood (always sea caught and never farmed). Here's a good guide when it comes to getting adequate quality proteins that count.

HIGHESTPROTEINS

Turkey
Snapper
Clams
Beef
Tuna
Veal
Chicken livers
Chicken
Beef liver
Beef steak

MEDIUMLEVELPROTEINS

Eggs
Cheeses
Sausage
Nuts
Seeds

Proteins are also found in vegetables and legumes.

But remember, proteins are nothing without fats! You might like to learn that marrow and organ meats such as brains provide excellent sources of monosaturated and omega 3 respectively. If these foods aren't your cup of tea, you might like to include other excellent sources of fat including nuts, avocados and oils.

Instead of brains, you might choose to switch to seafoods, flaxseed oil, free range poultry, pasture fed, grass finished meats, eggs, nuts, green leafy veggies – all excellent substitutes and great sources of nutrients that your body requires to be healthy and maintain that lean physique.

How to order when dining out

At first it can seem daunting when eating out. A little practice makes perfect when it comes to the enjoyable job of choosing your food and keeping your awesome self in check!

When you look at a menu, always look for the whole foods, the way nature intended them to be. Foods that fall into these categories are the meats and fish, plants and seeds. Some dairy is okay here too – we're a huge fan of goat's dairy. Don't forget that pasta is heavily processed, as are bread and many fried foods.

To save yourself time and cravings, skip to the mains when eating out. You can generally choose from a great range of fish, meat or poultry based dishes with a delicious side serving of nourishing vegetables or salad to match.

If you really want to join in on the entrée action, find your paleo friendly options in fish dishes like calamari or sardines. Olives, suitable cheeses and antipasto platters are also very friendly options.

It's quite simple to enjoy dining out and not missing out!

A word on grains

Grains are a staple part of the modern diet. But in ancient times, they weren't readily available as we see them today and therefore they weren't part of a Paleolithic diet. The biggest problem with many modern grains is that they are most often highly processed and often incomplete – meaning we are only eating part of the grain and not the whole food.

What's more, through genetic modification, they look quite different from the way nature intended them to be. For some, they can be difficult to digest and often contain gluten. Most grains and legumes also contain high levels of phytic acid, which binds minerals and eliminates them from the body leading to iron, calcium, magnesium and zinc deficiency.

Legumes, whilst they contain protein, these are incomplete proteins and can inhibit your body's ability to digest properly. Both grains and legumes also contain other substances which lead to a host of issues as they disrupt thyroid function leading to a swag of problems including mental and behavioural disorders and food allergies.

The good news is we can minimise and often remove phytic acid from grains by soaking them overnight before preparation. We've even got a recipe to show you how to sprout nuts. Sprouting or fermenting can also have the same effect and pump up the nutritional factor 10 fold. It must however be said that high consumption of carbohydrate isn't ideal - keeping it on the lower end of the scale is best.

With this in mind, some grains are more easily digested and acceptable than others. Ancient grains and those free from gluten may be ok in moderation depending on individual requirements and constitution. Such grains include quinoa, millet, spelt (although it contains gluten, it is easy for most to digest), amaranth, buckwheat and rice.

Much of your body's ability to digest grains will depend on several things like your blood type, your gut health and food combination. We advise that grains be consumed conservatively – there are some benefits to including grains in our diet. They provide fuel and easily accessible nutrition – they are readily converted in our bodies to energy. That said, the primary source of carbohydrate should still be from fruit and vegetables.

Ice age humans consumed little dietary fiber. However certain antioxidants and nutrients are found in fibrous vegetable and fruits and are of great value to the body. Such varieties of vegetables and fruits have been typically available in healthy primitive hunger-gatherer societies and their nutritional properties more important to us now than ever. Fibre however isn't the critical part of the nutritional equation - vegetables and especially high sugar fruits are not the cornerstone to a healthy diet.

Studies (and evolution) suggest that fibre from vegetables and fruits may not be as central to our health and longevity as nutritional pundits - excess dietary fibre can lead to these deficiencies we've previously discussed. Fibre, especially from grains can really irritate the colon.

However, soluble fibre found in nuts, seeds and fibrous vegetables and fruit can serve to support healthy gut bacteria - and the bacteria can convert the fibre into useful nutritional substances.

the best thing

about fibre is that it doesn't convert to sugar. So get into your veggies any way you can!

CHAPTER FIVE

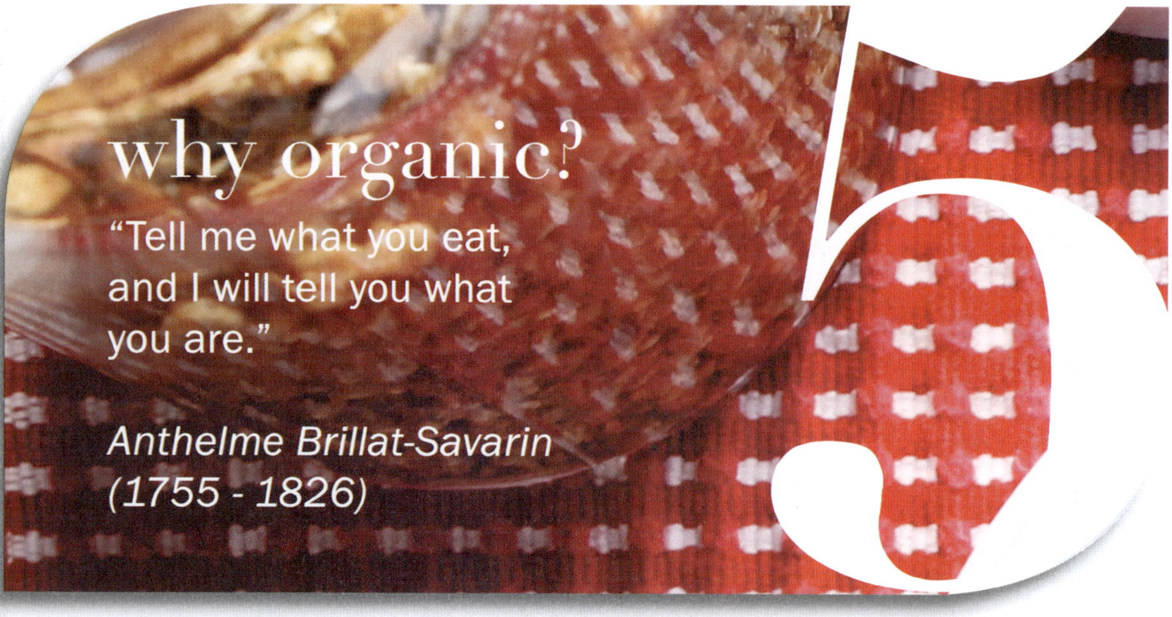

why organic?

"Tell me what you eat, and I will tell you what you are."

Anthelme Brillat-Savarin (1755 - 1826)

organic is the new black

Have you noticed how the label "organic" is starting to take over supermarket shelves?

It refers to foods produced in soils and environments that contain 5% of chemical residues and have no added pesticides or herbicides. Many people today are no longer willing to expose themselves and their children to what scientific research is revealing to be a widespread and growing pesticide health hazard. In fact, one major chain now has over 300 organic products, ranging from pasta to juice, canned foods, cereals, and even meat.

There are grocers and stores that specialise in organic produce popping up everywhere, and this is happening in response to increased public awareness and informed concern about the importance of nutrition. It is a growing and multi-million dollar industry for one reason only – demand. The demand for organic food has made it the new black in the food industry.

There was actually a time when the only food available was organic, because the chemicals didn't exist and food wasn't farmed the way it is now. People got their nutrition from food that was grown naturally and wasn't robbed of its vital minerals and nutrients.

What has happened to our eating habits? Our soils have been sterilised by the use of chemicals sprayed on produce. This is a major problem because much of the nutrients are passed from the ground where the plant is grown, into the plant. Our modern foods are so full of hormones and pesticides that the nutritional and mineral content is questionable. Food industry adulteration and devitalisation has created the growing need for vitamins and supplements as we just aren't getting the nutrition we require from conventional foods.

For example, nuts are 'bombed' as soon as they enter the country. Huge warehouses full of imported nuts are drenched with pesticide bombs so powerful that the doors must be sealed shut to prevent the poisons escaping into the atmosphere. We can't breathe it, so why would anyone think we can eat it?

Organic food is so much more appealing nutritionally and tastes unbelievably different. It is a little more costly at the moment, but increased demand will inevitably bring an equalisation in price as more primary producers enter this increasingly lucrative market. And keep in mind that what you are presently saving short-term in dollars by buying adulterated foods, you are losing long-term in the negative effects on your mind and body.

Eating organically may sound a little daunting at first, but the best way to start is with a monthly shopping trip to your local organic or farmers' market, which is usually very affordable. Open up your senses and give yourself time to explore this new environment. Walk around and observe the different products available, try some of the fresh fruit and vegetable juices and taste the difference. Notice the different size, colour, scent and 'feel' of the vital foods there. There are many organic food delivery services now too, so there's really no excuse.

Understand that the organic fresh produce may not always be as pretty as the waxed apples or sprayed broccoli you normally see in a supermarket. Remember, the pretty appearance is achieved only with the use of chemicals that may have the same effect on you as they did on the insects and other organisms they exterminated. Combine that with the likelihood that the apples and oranges you buy have potentially been in storage for up to eight months. And it doesn't stop there. All produce at your local supermarket has been stored away. It's a nutritional disaster.

Broccoli is one of the most sprayed foods, so to make a big difference in your wellbeing you might like to start with the organic variety of this delicious vegetable. It will not only taste much better, but it could end up saving you money in the long run as you appreciate it more, eat less, and require less supplementation.

Some organic foods may even surprise you with a worm lurking around in there. They may startle, but they won't harm you, and as long as you thoroughly wash the organic food, it's fine. Bugs are actually a guarantee of quality, because most insects cannot survive in foods that have been chemically treated, so if it's good enough for the worm to eat, it's okay for you as well.

You should actually be more worried that you don't find any worms on your normal food, as the harsh chemicals on the sprayed food have driven away or killed them. What do you think the pesticide will do to you? The main thing is that if you are going to invest in eating organic, it too has to be fresh.

Is organic food healthier for us?

The exact nature and degree of the benefits of eating organic food have yet to be subjected to rigorous research, but anecdotal evidence abounds. At the very least, organic foods improve health because fewer pesticides, herbicides, waxes, and chemical fertilisers are used than with non-organic foods.

So is all organic food by definition a guarantee of health and reliability? No, unfortunately even here you must remain discriminating and continue to take responsibility for your own wellbeing. The meat in an organic sausage may be free of antibiotics, but it can still be high in saturated fat, which raises your cholesterol levels and affects your heart.

Similarly, some organic biscuits and cakes may contain a lot of refined sugars which can lead to problems such as obesity, as well as some preservatives and additives (although the Soil Association and other regulatory bodies permit only a few). So let moderation be your guide with both organic and non-organic foods, and choose foods that don't come in packets. Packaged foods usually have preservatives. Preservatives preserve.

Organic food is more natural, tastier and helps keep you away from 'fast' and processed foods. This is because there is a part of the brain that recognises the higher nutritional content and switches off the hunger mechanism sooner. It feels more satiated from nutrition than volume. An example is tomatoes. You need to eat 100 conventional tomatoes to get the same nutrition as one organic one.

Not only is organic food more nutritious, it reduces your intake of dubious and harmful chemicals that can have lasting negative effects on your health. Good food is not just healthy food; in many ways it can be a healing agent.

If you want more life, eat more live and organic foods.

Eat foods that are alive, not packaged – fresh fruit, vegetables and foods that grow.

When choosing more live foods in your diet consider adding sprouts. A sprout is the beginning of a vegetable, and will provide you with more energy as it is new life and is bursting with growth.

Broccoli (as we mentioned) and potatoes are often the most sprayed vegetables, so buy the organic versions.

Remember, if you don't like, or are not used to, eating vegetables, we recommend trying the organic varieties as they taste quite different and better. You may find that organic carrots or pumpkin are actually sweet. If you can't taste the difference, detox from coffee, cigarettes and other toxicities to remove the coating from your taste buds.

When juicing, the best type of juicer to use is one that squashes (masticates) the fruit or vegetable. The motor doesn't heat up like a regular juicer and kill off the essential nutrition and minerals in the food. Juicing the food in this type of juicer will maximise your mineral and nutritional intake.

Stay away from MSG (monosodium glutamate, 621). It is found in lots of packaged foods, is highly addictive and can make you hungrier. Although that will be the least of your worries; it is so toxic, it may also affect your mood and cause depression.

Most importantly, get rid of your microwave! As easy as it has become to cook and heat foods this way, you may as well be throwing your good organic food away; studies have found that microwaves may destroy many of your food's vital nutrients.

The doctor of the future

"The doctor of the future will give no medicine, but will interest his patients in the care of the human frame, in diet, and in the cause and prevention of disease."

Thomas Edison

Food is fuel

Imagine you have a Ferrari, or perhaps you already do. Would you put water, or dirt, or even regular fuel in the fuel tank? Of course not. In fact, you would use only top quality high-octane fuel to get the best performance and longest life from your beautiful machine, and reduce repair costs.

Well, your body is a Ferrari. It is unquestionably the most evolved, intricate, and powerful vehicle on the planet; a brilliantly designed self-healing and self-regulating machine that is using everything you put into it to recreate itself every minute of the day.

Putting poor quality or junk food in your body is exactly like putting inferior fuel in a Ferrari. Your body is so resilient that even with the worst food it will still produce cells and continue to function, but the long-term effects of empty, non-nutritious foods are devastating.

Eventually the body can no longer adapt or compensate, with the result being disease and accelerated aging. It's strange that we would take more care of a manmade machine than a divinely created one, but we do. So begin to think of your body as a Ferrari. Give it only the best fuel, and let it give you its best in return.

We are hopeful for a future where the history of medicine reads as follows:

"Doctor, I have an earache."

2000 B.C.	"Here, eat this root."
1000 B.C.	"That root is evil, say this prayer."
1850 A.D.	"That prayer is superstition, drink this potion."
1940 A.D.	"That potion is snake oil, swallow this pill."
1985 A.D.	"That pill is ineffective, take this antibiotic."
2000 A.D.	"That antibiotic is artificial and can harm you. Here, eat this root!"

There's validity in the saying "get back to your roots" for more reason than one. So far from our roots, and so far from being natural, is the notion that if we eat artificial sweetened foods then we will also lose weight.

(Extract from 7 Things Your Doctor Forgot to Tell You)

myth:

ARTIFICIALSWEETENERHELPSYOU LOSEWEIGHT

Artificial sweetener has been promoted as the great breakthrough for weight watchers because it is virtually calorie free. It's actually misleading. Even though it has no calories, it is a chemical that your body doesn't know how to digest, and by making it harder to process foods, actually slows down your digestive system, thereby causing weight gain. As unwelcome as that is, it is actually benign compared to its many other side effects.

Most foods that are labelled 'low fat' or 'light' will contain artificial sweetener, and again you may think you're losing weight or being healthier by eating less sugar or fat, but they may actually make you put on weight.

argh!

The effects go beyond this, because studies show that long-term use creates an environment for blood-borne cancers like lymphoma to develop. All this time we have been led to believe that we were making healthier choices when we opted for artificial sweeteners, just because they had fewer calories.

You're now getting an inkling of the possible dangers of regular aspartame consumption. There are countless reports and research from doctors and nutritionists who have 'cured' their clients of many conditions, simply by removing aspartame from their diets.

The multi-billion dollar aspartame industry would have us believe that "aspartame kills" is an urban legend, and that it would require the consumption of 100 cans of diet soda a day to be harmed by their product. Despite it being untrue that 'diet' drinks help you to lose weight, their main claim is that the three components of aspartame are found in many natural foods and are therefore safe. This is like saying that carbon monoxide is safe because it contains only carbon and oxygen, the same components as carbon dioxide.

The following report by Dr Felicity Lawrence further explores the controversy surrounding man-made artificial sweeteners.

Methanol (wood alcohol) makes up 10% of aspartame and is highly toxic - the minimum lethal dose for an adult is two teaspoons. It is also found in some fruits and vegetables, but never occurs in natural foods without ethanol and pectin, its 'antidotes'. Ethanol & pectin prevent methanol from being metabolised into formaldehyde (embalming fluid) & formic acid (the same chemical as fire ant venom), both deadly toxins. An ethanol drip is the standard emergency room treatment for methanol poisoning. Aspartame contains no ethanol or pectin; therefore the methanol is converted to formaldehyde and formic acid in your body when you consume it, which are toxic.

1. San Francisco Chronicle, January 2, 1970

The sickly sweet facts

Aspartame, the essential ingredient in many artificial sweeteners, breaks down to phenylalanine, aspartic acid, and methanol when heated, and also within our warm bodies. The methanol is further metabolised into formaldehyde, a poison known to damage the immune and nervous system as well as cause genetic damage.

Aspartame breaks down the protective coating surrounding neurons in our brain, causing a break in the blood-brain barrier and allowing toxins to move directly into the bloodstream, with a whole cascade of destructive effects.

About 10% of the population has a tendency to multiple sclerosis (MS) but never actually develop the symptoms, and these people can be pushed into full-blown MS with continual usage of products containing aspartame.

Almost half of aspartame by weight is itself a toxin, technically an excitotoxin (a substance that damages nerve cells). Research done on 1,800 rats showed that it causes cancer of the kidney and of the peripheral nerves in the head. Earlier data from the same study linked aspartame to a greater risk of leukaemia and lymphomas, even at doses very close to what is considered the acceptable daily intake for humans.

Obviously, with such a list of dangerous side effects, aspartame should never be given to children.

The study concluded that consuming products containing aspartame may contribute to ailments such as: birth defects, brain cancer, chronic fatigue, diabetes, dizziness, emotional disorders, epilepsy, Graves' disease, headaches, lowered sperm count, migraines, MS - multiple sclerosis and Parkinson's disease symptoms.

Another leading artificial sweetener is saccharin, which is popular because it is so much sweeter than sugar. It has been in use for longer than any other artificial sweetener and has been subjected to the most studies. When research linked it to cancer in 1977, it was not banned because there were no alternative sweeteners for diabetics at the time. The U.S. permitted its use as long as manufacturers affixed a warning label, so in that country many products like chewing gum bear the legend: "This product contains saccharin, which has been known to cause cancer in laboratory animals".

Cyclamate was also at one time a widely used artificial sweetener, but this chemical has been banned in the U.S. since 1970 based on its possible link with cancer.

Dr Joseph Mercola (www.mercola.com) has dedicated his life to revealing the truth behind artificial sweeteners, and has published the results of his research in the book Sweet Deception. This topic deserves a whole book on its own, so if you really want to know the facts this is an excellent source. It will shake any blind trust you might have in the authorities overseeing what is allowed to be added and done to our food, and give you a fuller understanding of just how decisions by organisations like the U.S. Food And Drug Administration (FDA) may be hazardous to your health.

In 1970, former FDA commissioner Charles Edwards said: "People think the FDA is protecting them. It isn't. What the FDA is doing and what the people think it's doing are different as night and day."(1)

In that instance he was referring to the fact that the FDA not only works to protect 'pharma-business', but also actively works against good health practices and has done so for years.

Note: *If you're diabetic, then you have good reason to seek alternate sweet sources, but choose wisely. There are many natural sweeteners that are much safer than any artificial ones, and once you reduce your sweets consumption, it's likely that your cravings will also abate.*

there are alternatives

Stevia and Xylitol vs. Sugar and Artificial Sweetener

Stevia is made from the leaves of the South American plant stevia rebaudiana. As a herb and a natural sweetener it is superior to any artificial product. Sweeter than regular sugar and with far fewer calories, it is used to sweeten tea in Japan and South America. Stevia is beneficial in balancing blood sugar, and has antimicrobial properties. Again, moderation is the key, but when such excellent herbal alternatives are available you needn't sweeten anything artificially.

Xylitol (dextrose) is another alternative to sugar and artificial sweeteners, and may be used safely in small amounts. Derived from the birch tree, it is widely used in chewing gums as it inhibits bacterial growth and reduces the incidence of cavities. It tastes exactly like sugar, and is especially good for diabetics and those who are hypoglycaemic. A 1986 study verified Xylitol's safety – it received the highest and safest ADI (acceptable daily intake) rating. You can purchase xylitol from health food stores and use it as a sweetener in drinks and baked goods.

It's a great sugar alternative and has 40% less calories than sugar. It's also plant-derived, which means it's natural, unlike aspartame, which has been known to be carcinogenic and affect the digestive system.

Agave nectar is also plant-derived and a great sugar alternative. The texture is more like syrup than thick honey. It makes it a great consistency for baking. There are 'lighter' versions of agave nectar, but the light type means it is only lighter in colour, not calories, so choose the darker amber colour, which has a rich, delicious flavour.

While no sweetener is without controversy, artificial sweeteners can be quite damaging to our health and may cause serious illness. If you have the choice, and you do, it's best to avoid them completely. Some people choose them because they've been led to believe that artificial sweetener is actually healthier and better for them than sugar. It is not. All artificial sweeteners are exactly that — artificial.

So you're already doing all the right things and exercising, right? What's wrong then? Well the key to unlocking 'thin' is to avoid sugar, eat good fats often, allow better nutritional value through eating organic and make sure your body can assimilate the great nutrition.

CHAPTER SIX

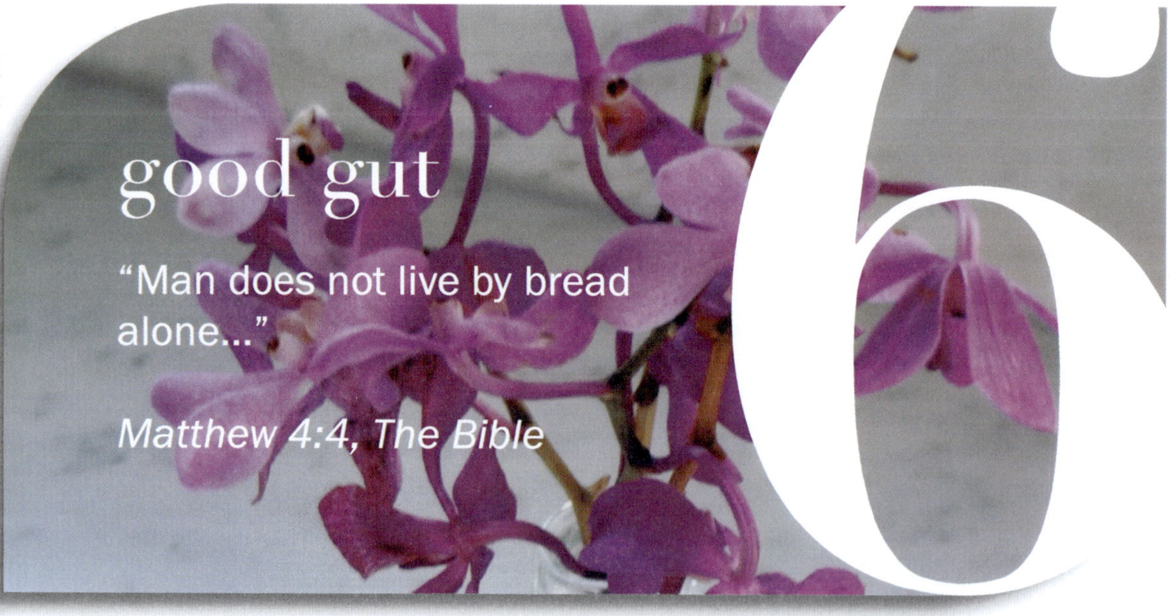

6 good gut

"Man does not live by bread alone..."

Matthew 4:4, The Bible

In fact, ditch the bread too!

Processed white bleached flour or even plain wheat can wreak havoc on your gut. Most of us are intolerant to gluten, some of us may not even realise it. It's this type of carbohydrate that causes a smorgasbord of issues like bloating, constipation, irritable bowel syndrome and even fertility and reproductive issues.

To better understand the gut, it may help if we break it down as to how it works. You may have heard of the term 'leaky gut' – when our foods dangerously leak into our systems and cause illness. Now, a normal, healthy gut is full of bacteria – some bad but mostly good. Bad bacteria, in full force can also cause troubles, but in most people, the good bacteria outweigh the bad and keep it under control.

Your gut lining is made up of these bacteria (approximately 3kg of it actually) which line your digestive tract from top to bottom. This bacteria acts as a barrier between your actual gut lining and your food. So imagine, from your mouth right through to your bowel, millions and trillions of little soldiers all lined the entire way through – always ready for action. These bacteria have a multitude of functions. They help digest your food and break down nutrients, allowing it to be distributed around your body to 'feed' it. This also helps shape your immunity as your body's ability to fight off pathogens is greater when we are in good health.

What's more, because of their ability to balance bacteria, they're always fighting off anything trying to invade your body. They also provide a protective layer to the gut and stop food from literally leaking into your body. Without these protectors, our guts can end up in a pretty terrible state.

We now know that antibiotics, overconsumption of alcohol and a poor diet will not only clear out bad bacteria in the event of illness but also the good bacteria. Without the good bacteria, the body loses its fighting power and is often left defenceless, especially after illness, which is why people often relapse or are repeatedly unwell – their body has lost its ability to fight for itself. See, your body really has much of what it requires to fight off illness. If we support it in the right way, there is very often little need for harmful medications.

Without all these little fighting soldiers forming a protective barrier, we are left helpless in the event of illness. As we've outlined, without a healthy gut, our bodies can't assimilate the nutrients from the foods we eat and redistribute it to feed the body. The process can't occur properly which is why our immune system takes a back seat.

As if our gut wasn't already clever enough, it is also full of receptors and nerves which largely play a role in our emotional health. You've probably felt sick in your gut before when you've received bad news or lost your appetite when you're sad. This is because of these receptors in your gut. We now know that our guts are like our second brain; they shape much of our body's ability to function.

Without a healthy gut you may see skin conditions, irritable bowel, gynaecological disorders including fertility issues and thrush – we could keep going all day because almost all health problems can be related back to poor digestive and gut function. But the good news is that you can repair a damaged gut.

The foods you eat and the lifestyle you lead are key in maintaining and re-establishing healthy gut function. Some bacteria can take up to 16 months to re-grow following illness and the use of antibiotics. Some bacteria, unless action is taken, will never grow back after the use of antibiotics. This is bad news for people who are unaware of the damage antibiotics are doing to our bodies.

But the good news is there are specific foods that help to repair and heal the gut. These include pro-biotic and fermented foods, a diet rich in therapeutic fats including those found in fish, coconut oil, nuts, seeds, avocado – all the foods we here at Eat Fat, Be Lean love most. Not only are they good for your gut, they also tick boxes in every area of supporting wellness.

Pro-biotic foods can be tricky to get your hands on. In Australia, we have very strict laws that prevent unpasteurised foods from being sold. Problem is, it is the unpasteurised nature of such foods that hold the pro-biotic content. Probiotic and fermented foods were once a part of our staple diet. We didn't have fridges, so we had to pickle and ferment foods to ensure they lasted through the off seasons. But in doing so, such foods were actually essential in maintaining health – they were high in probiotics.

You may have heard of these foods including sauerkraut, kifier yoghurt, Korean kim-chi or fermented tea known as kombucha. Including these in your diet, you are always topping up these gut bacteria. For those who are lacking specific bacteria, these are your ticket to wellness, the key to a healthy gut.

The best way to get your hands on probiotic foods is to make them yourself. That jar of sauerkraut you found at the supermarket may be tasty, but it will not contain the necessary nutrients and probiotic properties due to those strict laws preventing unpasteurised foods being sold. Some health food shops do sell probiotic foods or the kits for you to make them at home. We have some suggestions in our shopping directory in the back of this book.

Fermenting your own foods

There are a variety of fermented foods you can make – these are our favourites as they are super simple.

KIFERYOGHURT

You can make it with coconut milk or dairy milk. It's as simple as adding the culture to milk and allowing to ferment (12 – 24 hours). You can obtain the culture online.

KOMBUCHA–FERMENTEDTEA

You'll need to obtain the bacteria or 'scoobie' online. It's as easy as making several cups of tea with a little sugar added (so that it can ferment), using a ceramic dish, adding the tea and the scoobie and left to do it's thing. The bacteria will sit on top and act like a 'seal' over the tea. Left to sit for 3 weeks or so, and you'll soon have your tea! Just be sure to submerse the scoobie regularly to keep the process coming along. You can use the scoobie over and over again.

Steps to a healthy gut

Add probiotics to your diet. Start slowly though as there is a period of time when you first add such foods called 'die off.' Die off is pretty self explanatory. It's when all those good bacteria go to work and battle it out with the bad guys. You may feel a little flu-like in this time if your gut health is particularly poor.

We suggest starting with a teaspoon of such foods and slowly increasing. You may like to do this over several weeks until you are able to have a serve per day, especially those who know they have poor gut bacteria presence.

Adding up the protein and fats is key to a top notch functioning gut. We've already outlined the importance of organics, adequate balance of proteins, and just how necessary fat is in your diet.

beware overconsumption of alcohol, medications and a poor lifestyle. Burning the candle at both ends just won't do. Be mindful to be having adequate R&R. **The best rule is 8 x 8 x 8.** That is 8 hours of sleep, 8 hours of work and 8 hours of play. Every day. Sleep is the elixir of good health. Those hours before midnight are worth double the value of those achieved after midnight. Cinderella was onto something! Aim to be in bed by 11pm each night for maximum benefits.

We've touched on the gut and emotional health – but stress is a huge factor in gut health. The combination of stress and gluten can send people running... literally! Not only that, stress can, for some, cause massive weight gain.

So in a nutshell – be aware of your lifestyle, emotional health, your diet and your environment and work out what specifically works for you body. This is the key to improved health and wellness.

How fat helps the gut

As we've established, fat is an essential part of a well balanced diet. In fact, so much so, we suggest that you grab the old school food pyramid you are well familiar with and flip it upside down! Hopefully you now understand that without therapeutic fats in your diet, our bodies simply can't function as our genetics require.

Fat is essential for survival. Fat nourishes our cells, it helps support that good gut bacteria and shape our immunity. Specific fats like coconut oil help to increase metabolism, improve circulation, repair cells and improve general health and wellbeing.

CHAPTER SEVEN

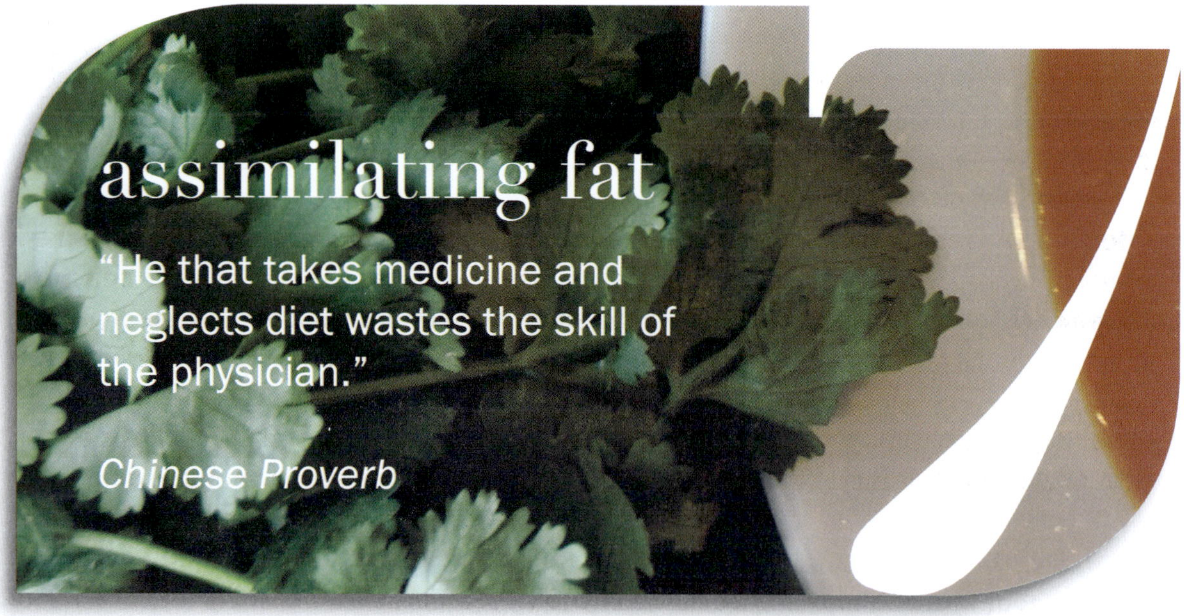

assimilating fat

"He that takes medicine and neglects diet wastes the skill of the physician."

Chinese Proverb

If you just gave birth to a beautiful new baby, you would want to fuel him with the best nutrients available, right? You wouldn't dream of feeding him chemicals or food scraps that were mouldy or put him at any risk of sickness. You might feel your body is too far gone if it needs some serious work and you have spent years abusing it. You might think it doesn't matter what kind of food you feed it. The reality is, it is never too late to start fuelling your body properly, and when it is well cared for and fed, it can assimilate food so much better – it's like brand new again.

This is where optimal health comes into play. Achieve optimal health by making the right choices to invest in your health. The World Health Organisation (WHO) states that health isn't merely the absence of disease or symptoms: it's also important to have optimal function.

WHO definition:

Health is a state of complete physical, mental, and social wellbeing and not merely the absence of disease or infirmity.

Complementary health care

CHIROPRACTICCARE

Chiropractic care can help with assimilation of fat and improve the digestive system. It's through your nervous system that you perceive the world, adapt to stress and coordinate all body functions. Making sure that your nervous system is free of interference will mean that there is a clearer signal from brain to body. You can achieve this clearer communication by being regularly checked by a wellness chiropractor who understands this.

Doctors of Chiropractic focus on removing nerve system interference by aligning the spine. It's the bones of the spine and the skull that protect the brain, spinal cord and nerves that branch off. Your nervous system is your master controller, so it's paramount for good health. Chiropractors are the only health professionals in the world trained to detect and correct vertebral subluxation (interferences to the nerve system).

You will need messages firing from your brain, down the spinal cord and nerves, in the healthiest possible way. Nerves tell muscles what to do. They're a reactive tissue, not an active tissue, meaning they don't have a mind of their own. They get told what to do by the nervous system. When you remove nerve system interference with chiropractic adjustment, by aligning the spine which protects your nerves, you may be taking pressure off nerves that are trying to send healthy signals to your digestive system.

It's very common for those with already healthy diets and active lifestyles who can't shift weight, to start to lose weight with chiropractic care. The same nerves that go to your lower spine for example, also branch off to your digestive system and reproductive organs for example. Having a chiropractic adjustment may be like taking the pressure off a hose pipe. Suddenly the messages to those organs, which are muscles too, are free flowing! You may experience better bowel elimination or a healthier metabolism.

Find a chiropractor that uses an objective measure of health. They may call themselves 'wellness chiropractors' and use the latest in technology like an EMG (electromyography) scan which is non-invasive and detects nerve system interference. This will help you to see which nerves are not working well and also measure your progress on a functional and structural level too, not just symptomatic.

To find your local chiropractor, call this toll free number for the Chiropractor's Association of Australia: 1800 075 003.

ACUPUNCTURE

Acupuncture is beneficial for all body systems, especially the digestive system. It works to maximise fat absorption and balance hormones. Just as your chiropractor might work on your spine to get the best out of your body, acupuncture works in a similar manner by encouraging and supporting healthy body function, influencing and encouraging nutrient and blood flow. The gut is the pivot of your health; if it is working to its best ability, everything follows suit. Your bowels will be happy, your immunity strong, you will be fertile and you will glow.

When there is illness in the digestive system, every inch of your body suffers. Acupuncture and herbal supplementation can be extremely useful in getting healthy gut function back on track, as it assesses why it's not working adequately and sets about helping the body correct itself rather than forcing it to happen.

Taking a pill to treat digestive issues such as irritable bowel or leaky gut only provides a band-aid solution. The minute you stop taking it, you're back to where you started — sick and tired. When we take the time to get our body to work properly again, there is no need to take medicine long term and the result isn't just a happy tummy, it's a happy body.

With this in mind, we know that if the gut is working properly, it's absorbing nutrients well. You now know that one of the most vital things your body requires to function optimally is fat. So if your gut is in tip-top shape, it will be able to use these dietary fats in such a way that your system can only thrive.

The same goes for your hormone balance. We see issues arise hormonally when there is inadequate fat intake, because our hormones are primarily made up of fats and protein. Without adequate fat, there simply isn't enough sustenance to make quality hormones. Hormones aren't limited to your reproductive system; they are present in all systems within your body, meaning they are vital for overall wellness.

Let's take this one step further and talk fertility for a second. Don't freak out at the F word – fertility. Being fertile doesn't necessarily equate to having a baby pronto. It's simply the ability to conceive; having a healthy reproductive system firing on all cylinders. With infertility rates rapidly climbing, it's imperative we recognise this link between healthy living and wellness. Our bodies aren't silly. If we aren't healthy, it knows to switch off the systems that aren't imperative to survive.

Your reproductive system is in the firing line here, because we can survive without it, at least for now. Should you be somebody who is experiencing menstrual issues, or is reproductively challenged, there is a good chance that making some positive lifestyle changes, including adding fat to your diet and shutting the door on gluten, will have a largely positive impact on your fertility.

Low fat dairy has been linked to infertility. A research project at the Harvard School of Public Health in Boston found that women who ate low fat and/or no fat dairy foods and no whole fat had 85% high risk of infertility – most commonly linked to an inability to produce healthy eggs.

If you're moving away from milk, then you may find that goat's milk or cheese can be better than cow's dairy. It's the protein in cow's dairy called casein that is too big for the human gut to digest. Your body creates extra mucous to balance the extra acid that is required to break down such a large and difficult-to-digest animal protein. However, the protein in goat's cheeses and milk is much smaller, and most people find they are not intolerant to this alternative.

When your body is working in harmony, you can rest assured that the fats you consume are being used and processed in the best way your body knows how.

Remember this – fat fills you up, making you eat less, full stop. Sugar doesn't. So you won't ever overeat fat. You will, however, overeat sugar as we have no 'off switch' when it comes to being full on the bleached white stuff. That means you won't get fat from eating fat. You will only get full.

Make sure your body is in tip-top healthy shape and functioning at its best with chiropractic and Chinese medicinal philosophies. It's the best weight-loss secret around.

BODYBUILDER'S BREAKFAST

Serves 4

Ingredients

- [illegible]
- [illegible]
- [illegible]
- [illegible]
- [illegible]
- [illegible]
- [illegible]
- [illegible]

Method

[illegible]

[illegible]

CHAPTER EIGHT

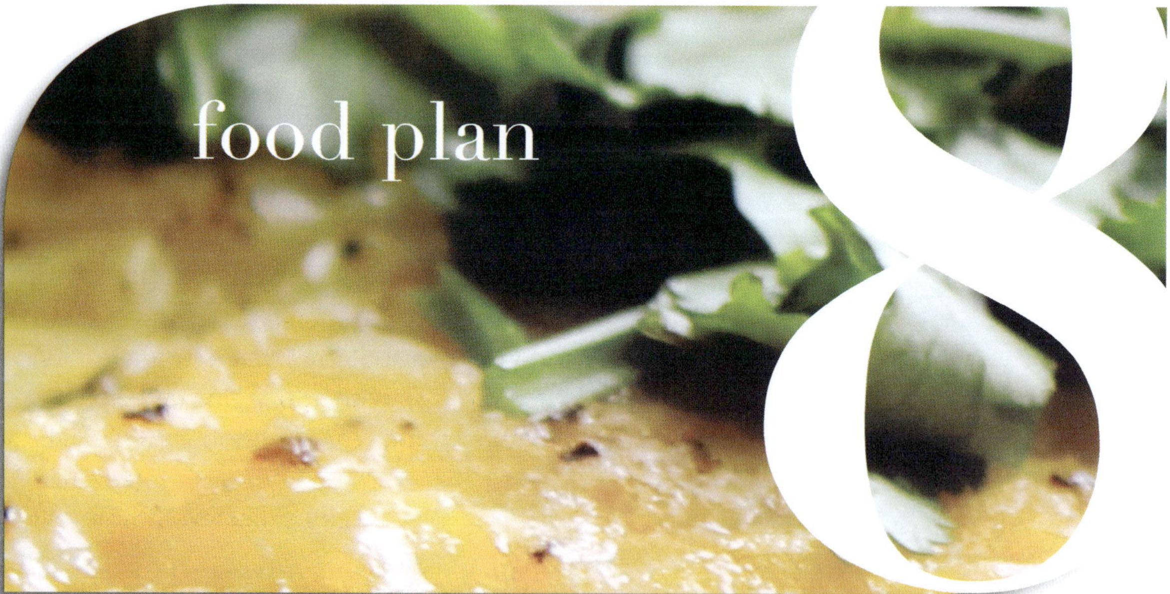

Start getting used to eating your new, good fats with every meal by getting ideas with our food plan example below. You may like to begin by writing down what you eat for a few weeks until you get the hang of it and can free ride. “Look mum! No hands!”

We want to hold your hand every step of the way, so feel free to stay in touch and ask questions about food alternatives or share with us how your baking went, as you go. We’d also love to hear about your results and changes you have discovered in your health and body.

You can keep in touch via our Facebook page Eat Fat, Be Thin – Sugar Free, Wheat Free, Dairy Free Recipes. Click ‘Like’ and stay connected or go to www.eatfatbethin.com.au for all our latest news and healthy sweet treats too. You may like to get a copy, if you haven’t already and start baking too.

Enjoy your food, protein fats and figures!

Be well. Live well. Move well.

love & *respect*

ANDI LEW AND DR NATALIE KRINGOUDIS

	breakfast	snack
1	Avocado and goat's cheese with scrambled eggs	Activated nuts and seeds
2	Scrambled eggs made with almond milk and smoked salmon	Poached pear and yoghurt sprinkled with Forage gluten-free cereal
3	Orange Chia Seed Cake from Eat Fat, Be Thin book	Veggie sticks and hummus
4	Forage Paleo Cereal	Carrot and Walnut Cake
5	Forage Rhubarb Crumble from Eat Fat, Be Thin book with a dollop of sheep's yoghurt	Salsa, tahini and corn chips

lunch	snack	dinner
Salmon steak and veggies	Sheep's yoghurt and blueberries	Gluten-free burrito (with beans or meat) with salsa and avocado
Japanese style hot pot	Amazeballs from Eat Fat, Be Thin book	Coconut milk fish and veggies
Lentil burger pattie with a huge salad	Miso soup	Bolognaise (meat or grated hard tofu) with gluten-free pasta
Meat or tofu Bolognaise with alkalising dark greens like spinach or shredded kale and gluten-free pasta	Goat's feta and olives	Thai-style stir fry with brown rice
Antipasto platter and vegetable soup	Coconut and pumpkin soup	Roast veggies with your choice of protein

Adequate water consumption is a vital part of healthy eating habits. As a guide, eight glasses per day will have your body happy – your skin benefits from this too as you are hydrated and nourished.

*Green tea is great for helping to break down fats and is a bumper of an antioxidant.

*As a rule, each meal should contain enough protein, which is enough to roughly fit the size of your hand.

This meal plan can be used for vegetarians and vegans too. Exchange fish or meat for beans, legumes, quality tofu and eggs.

CHAPTER NINE

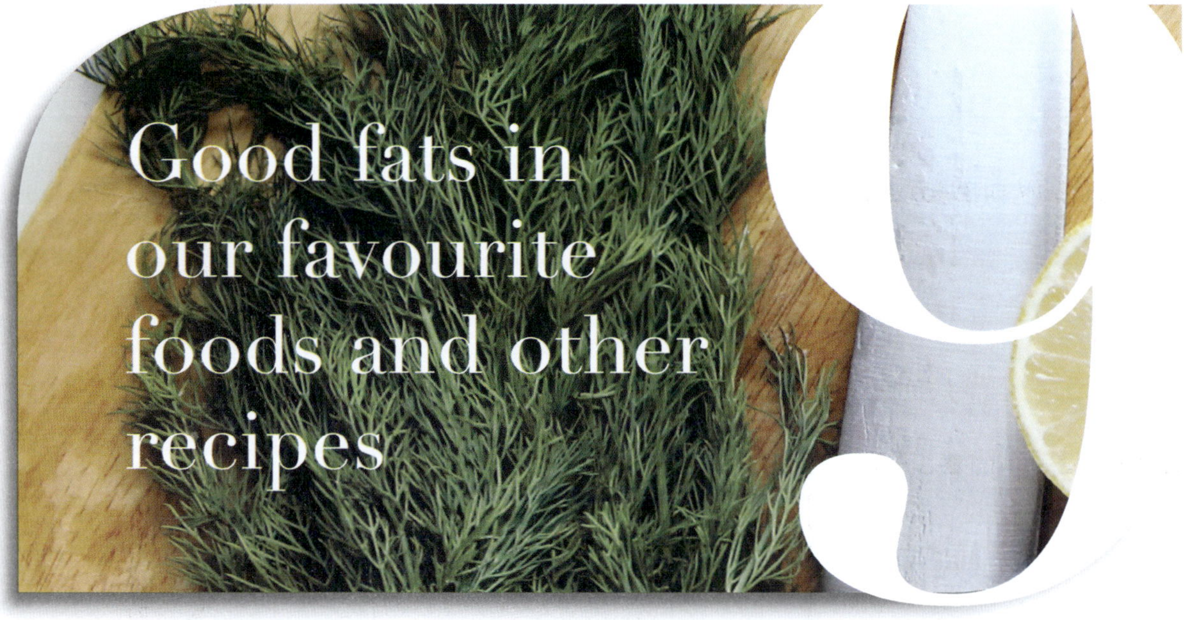

9 Good fats in our favourite foods and other recipes

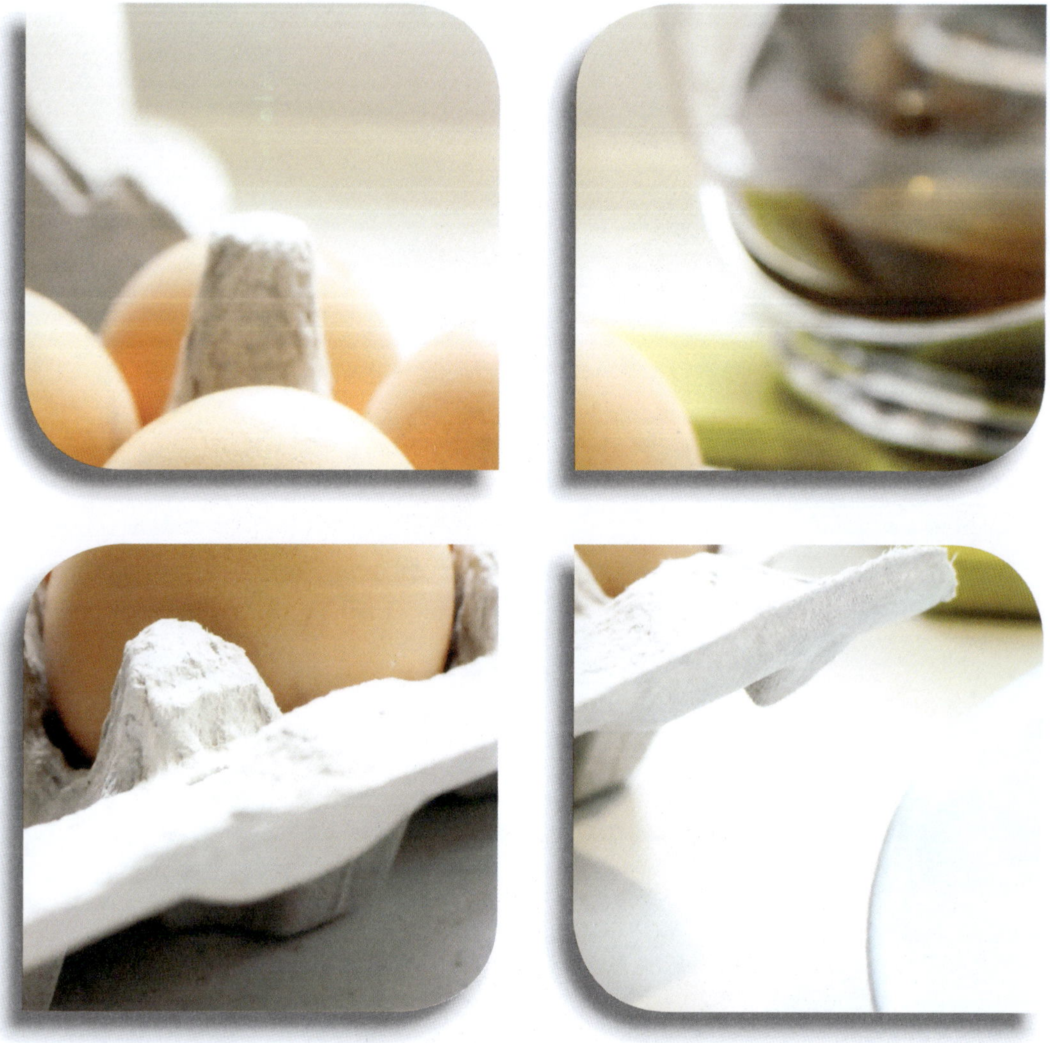

BREAKFASTS

BREAKFASTBURRITOS

These are so good and definitely not limited to breakfast time!

Serves 6

Ingredients

6 eggs
1 large red capsicum, sliced down the centre and then into thirds
Large handful of spinach
12 mushrooms, cut in half
12 cherry tomatoes cut in half
Coconut butter to grease muffin tray

Method

With coconut butter, grease each cup of a muffin tray
Arrange capsicum around one side of muffin cup
Across the other side, lay spinach to form a base
Crack 1 egg in each cup
Add mushroom and tomatoes evenly between cups
Season with salt and pepper
Place in a moderate oven, and bake until egg is cooked to your liking (approx 20-30 minutes)
Serve with avocado salsa.

BREAKFAST BURRITOS

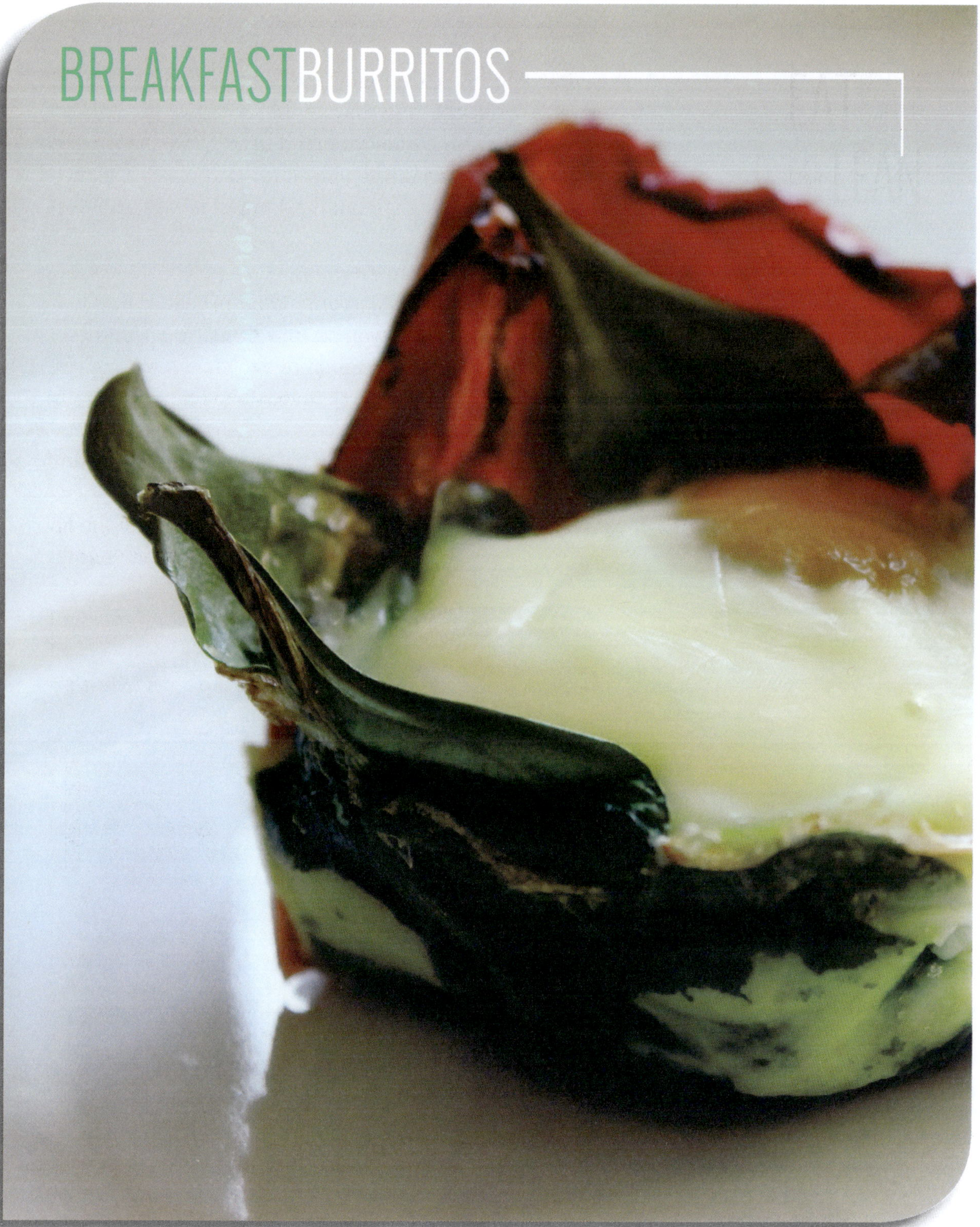

BODYBUILDER'S BREAKFAST

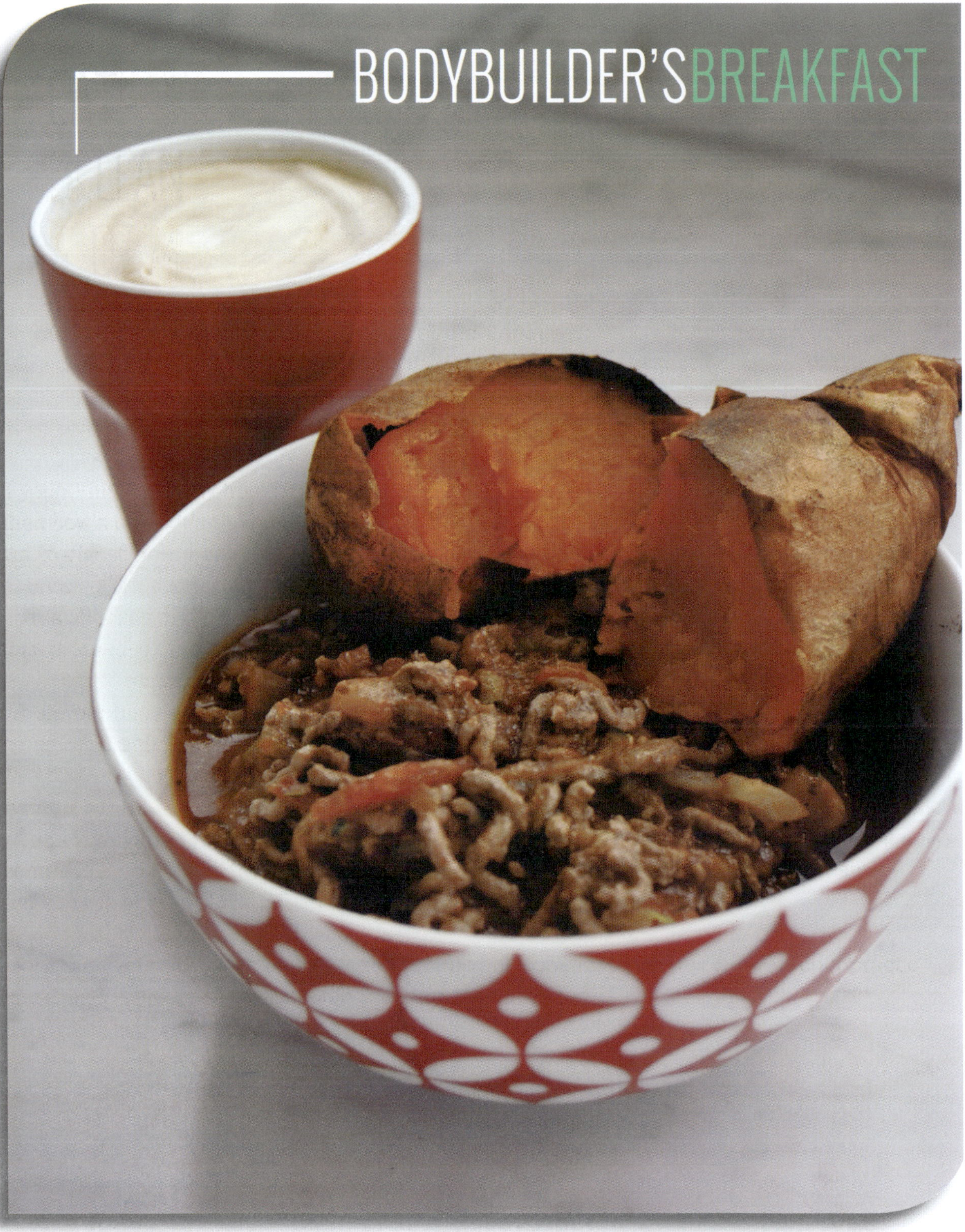

BODYBUILDER'SBREAKFAST

Serves 4

Ingredients

Minced organic beef (500g)
1 brown onion
1 large grated zucchini
1 packet of spinach leaves
1 jar of tomato pasta sauce without additives or preservatives
2 tbls of concentrated tomato paste
Sea salt
1 tbls coconut oil

Method

Fry the onion, chopped in a pan with the oil and brown, then add meat and zucchini to brown. Next add spinach and tomato pasta sauce. These usually contain basil. Make sure yours doesn't have sugar in it. Organic varieties are best or make your own with tomato puree and fresh herbs from your garden! Add a few sprinkles of sea salt and tomato paste, and let simmer for 6 mins.

Serve immediately or store and heat the next day in a pan. Do not reheat in microwave ovens as they may kill the nutritional content.

QUICKCHIASEEDPUDDINGS

Serves 2

Ingredients

1/2 cup of chia seeds
1 & 1/2 cups of cashew or almond milk (or regular milk if you so choose)
1/4 cup berries
Stevia to taste
1/2 teaspoon of vanilla powder
Pinch of salt

Method

Place all ingredients in a bowl and stir. Divide into bowls or containers and store in the fridge. You will need to allow it to absorb the liquid - the chia will take on a glutenous consistency (even though they are gluten free).

QUICK CHIA SEED PUDDINGS

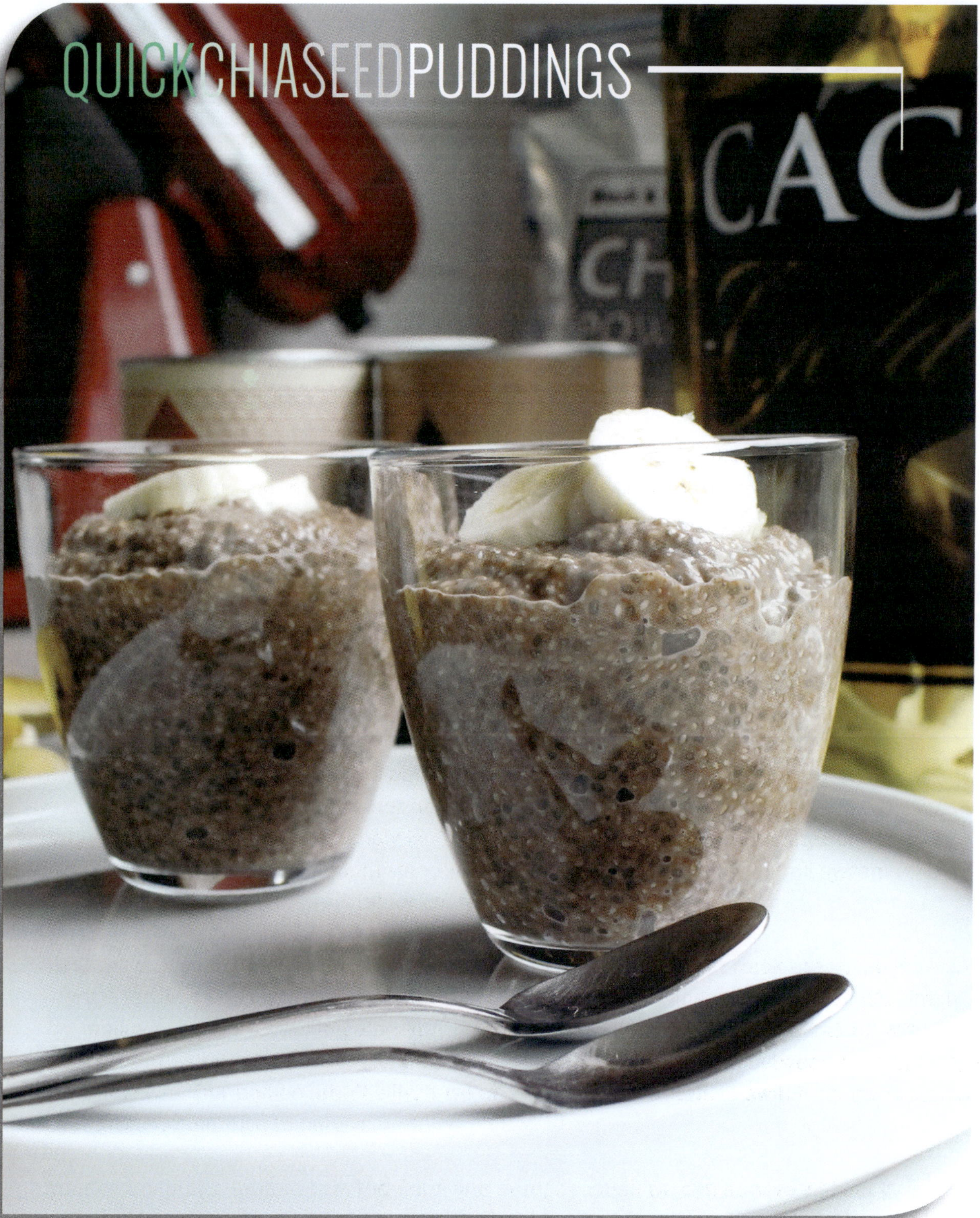

POACHED EGGS WITH TOMATO SALAD

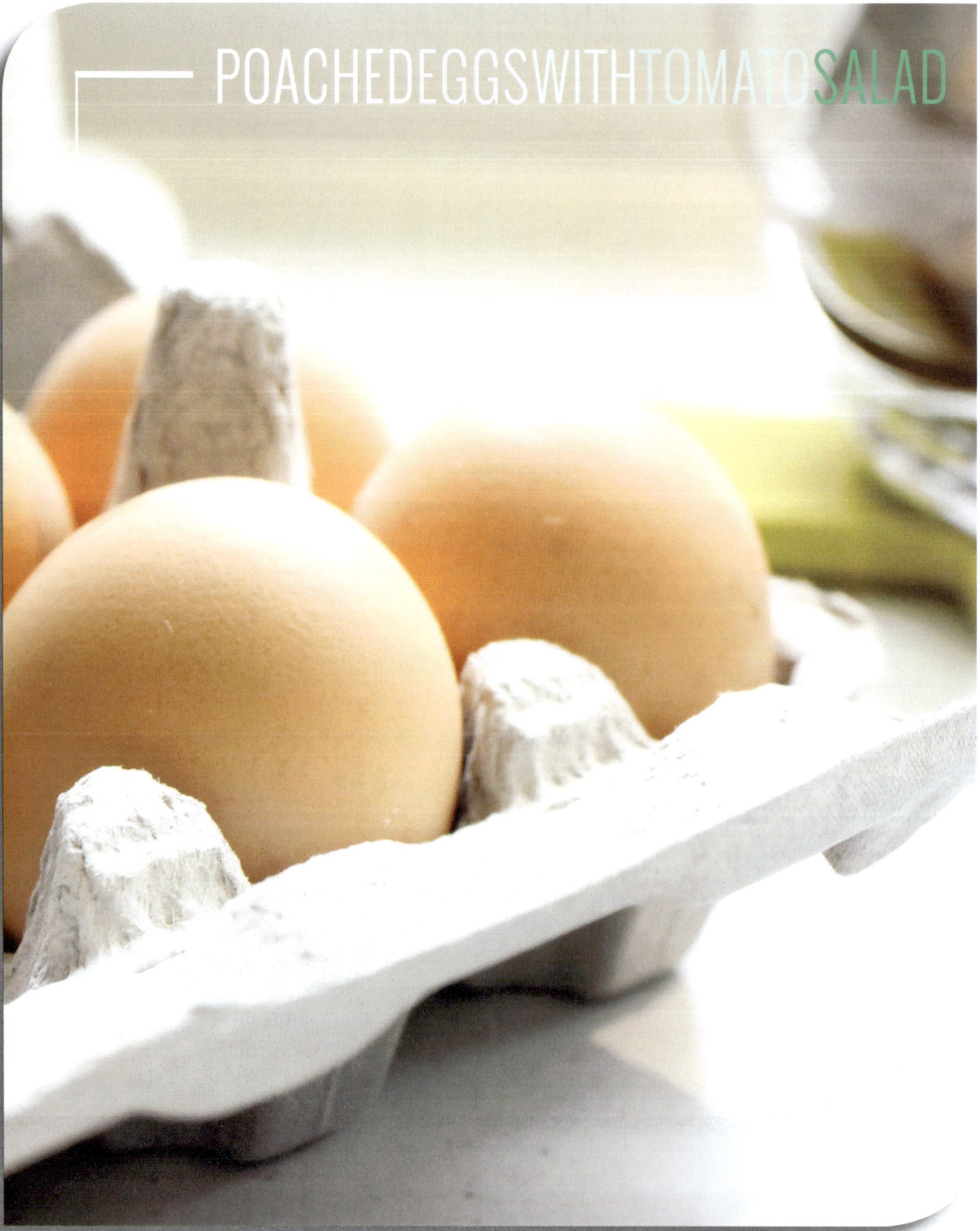

POACHEDEGGSWITH TOMATOSALAD

Serves 1

Ingredients

2 eggs
Boiling water to poach
Vinegar
2 tomatoes
1 avocado
Several basil leaves
Olive oil
Salt and pepper

Method

Boil water (approx 2-3 cups). Once boiled add a capful of vinegar to assist in the poaching process.

Stir the boiling water to create a currant and crack the eggs in, one by one.
Allow to cook to your liking.

To prepare the tomato salad, chop tomatoes, avocado, basil leaves and combine. Drizzle with olive oil and a dash of vinegar and season with salt and pepper before tossing.

GLUTENFREEGRANOLA

Makes 10+ serves

Ingredients

5 cups of forage
3 cups of chopped walnuts
1 cup chopped mixed nuts
1/2 cup of sunflower seeds
1/2 cup almond meal

In a separate bowl, place:

1 cup of the stewed apple – mashed
1 cup of the liquid left from the stewing process
3 tbls of coconut oil (or similar)

Method

Combine the two bowls - add the liquid to the dry ingredients and mix well adding more liquid if necessary (stewed liquid). Line two trays with baking paper and divide mixture between the two, then place into a 180°C oven and bake for 40 - 50, stirring every 10 minutes until mixture is completely golden and begins to dry out and harden.

Remove from oven and mix through dried fruit of your choice. I chose to chop dates and add currants.

Enjoy with milk as a breakfast or dessert.

GLUTEN FREE GRANOLA

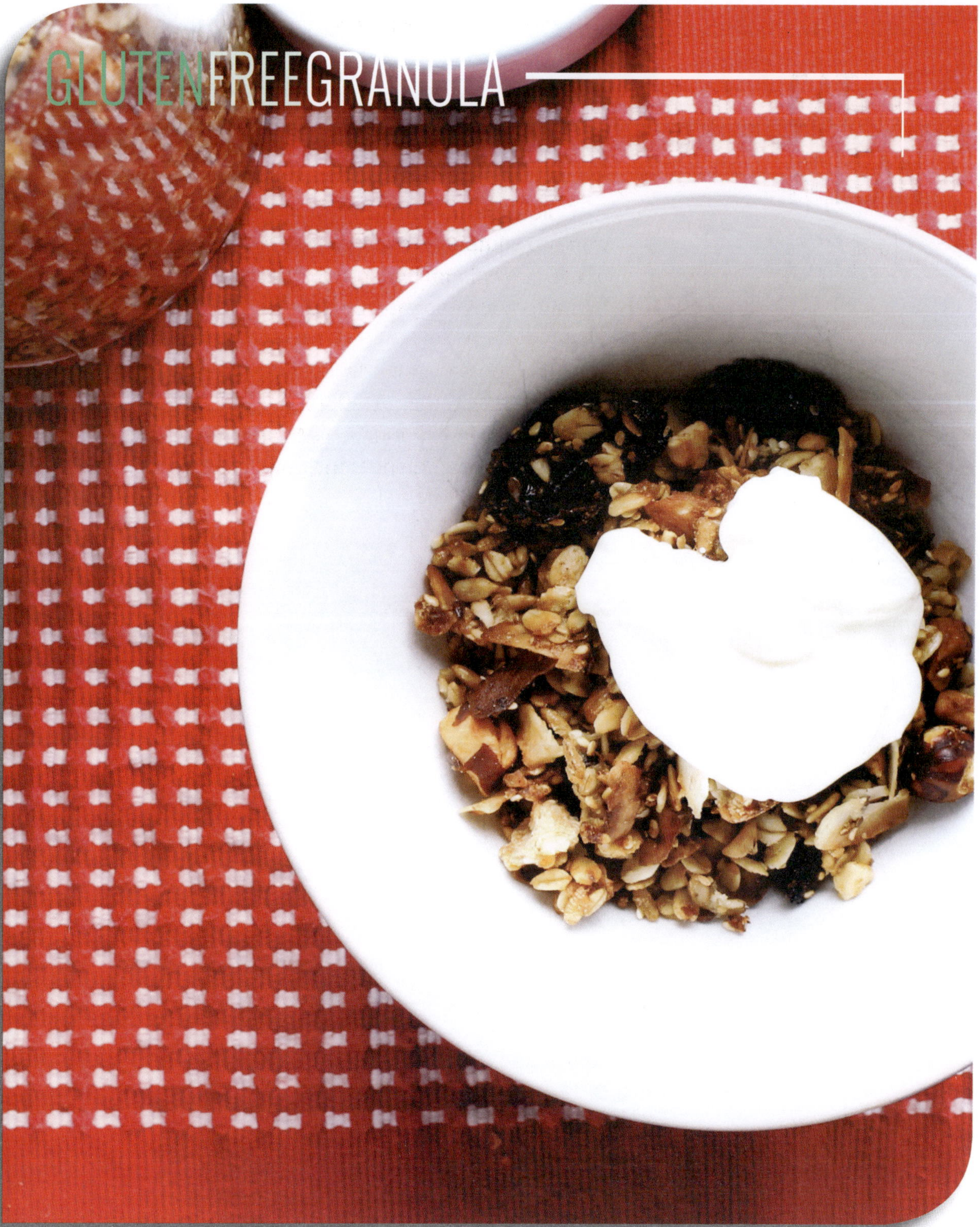

FORAGEPALEOCEREAL

This high fat cereal is totally unprocessed and includes:

Sunflower seeds
Cranberries
Almonds
Dates
Coconut
Pepitas
Currants
Pecans
Macadamia nuts

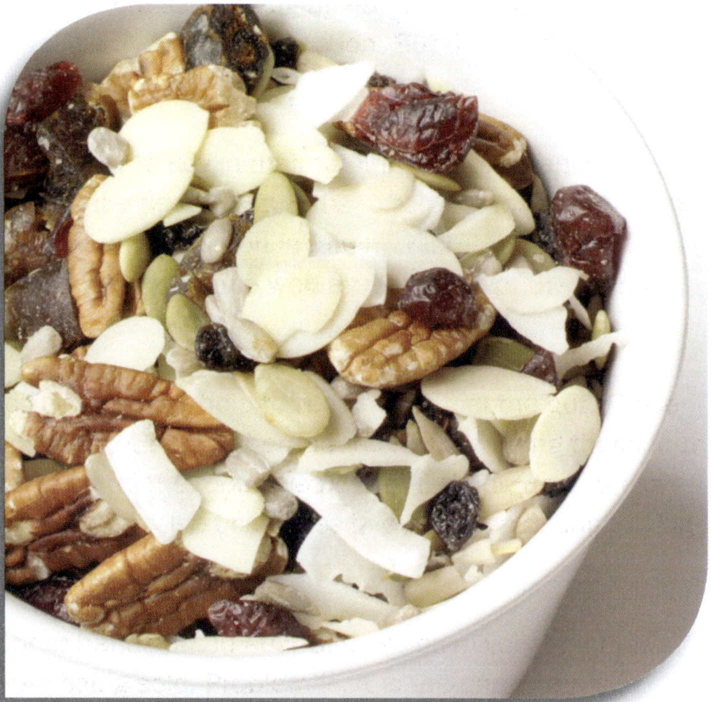

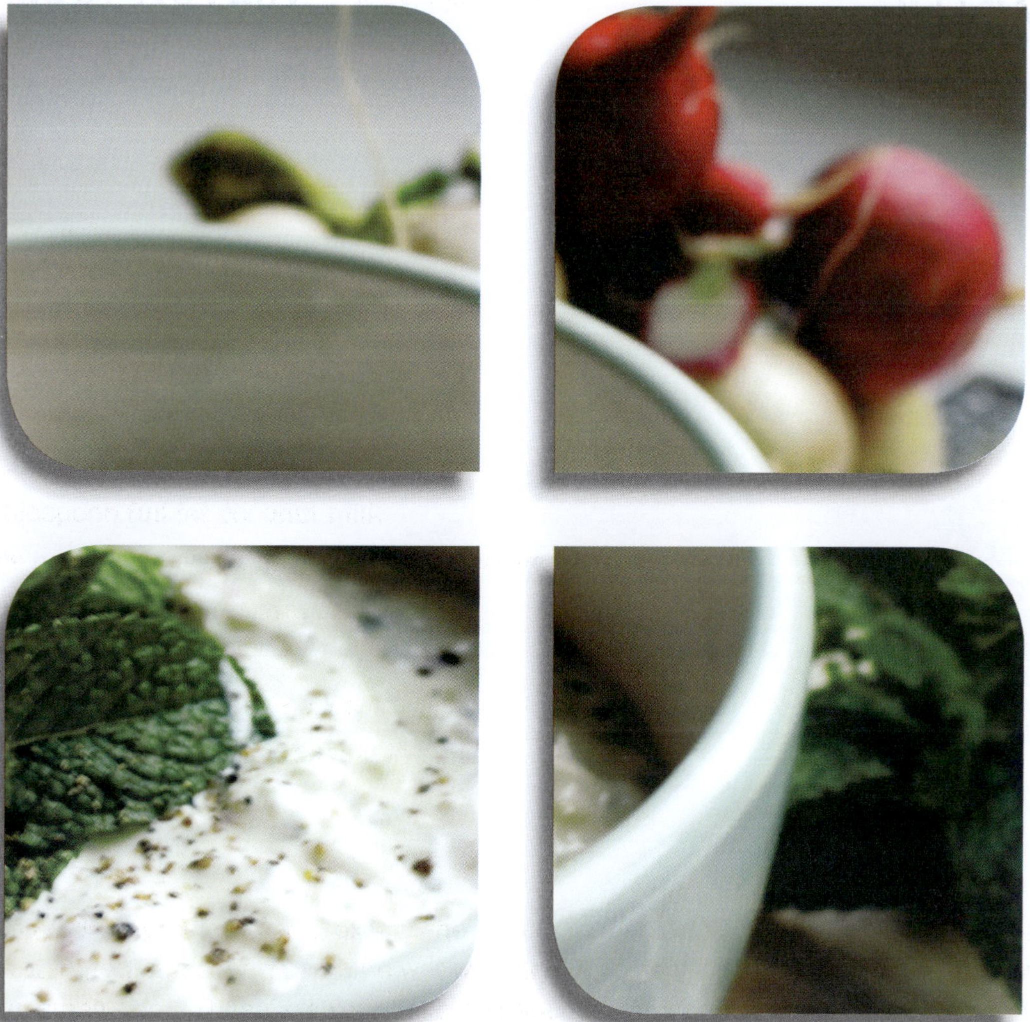

SNACKS

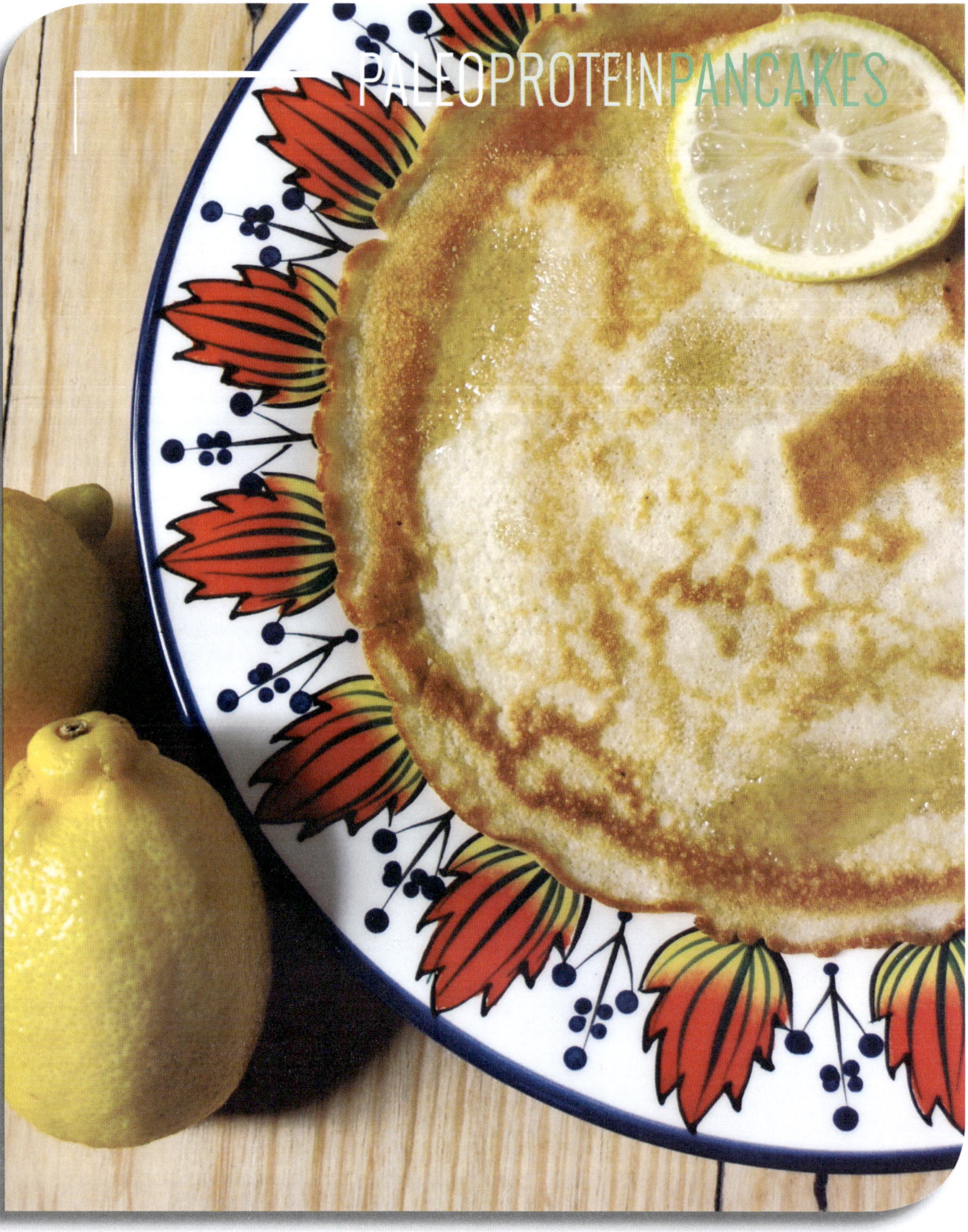
PALEOPROTEINPANCAKES

PALEOPROTEINPANCAKES

Serves 4

Ingredients

1 cup almond or hazelnut meal flour

½ teaspoon baking soda

¼ teaspoon sea salt

3 tablespoon full fat coconut milk

1 tbls honey or 2 drops of vanilla naturally sweet stevia

½ teaspoon of vanilla extract

Zest of ½ lemon

2 large organic, free-range eggs

1 tbls spoon coconut oil for frying in pan

Method

Combine dry ingredients first, except the lemon zest, in one bowl and in another bowl, mix the wet ingredients. Then combine wet with dry ingredients. Fold in lemon zest. Fry on a pan, small sizes. These are very delicate pancakes so cook them one at a time and in smaller sizes so they're easier to flip.

Serve warm with organic maple syrup and shredded coconut.

SPICYAVOCADOSALSA

Serves 4

Ingredients

3 ripe avocados
Sea salt
4 large organic tomatoes or 8 cherry tomatoes
2 shallots or half a purple onion
Lemon or lime juice
Fresh red chilli
Cracked black pepper

Method

Scoop out the avocados into a mixing bowl. Chop tomatoes and onion and chilli into small pieces. If you do not like very hot food, remove the chilli or at least the seeds from the chilli as this is where the heat is stored and will give flavour with less heat.

Mash the avocado with a fork. Let it stay chunky. Do not over mash. Then add the above ingredients and gently mix through, being careful not to mash the tomatoes. Squeeze fresh lime or lemon juice, add salt and pepper to taste.

Serve with vegetable sticks.

SPICY AVOCADO SALSA

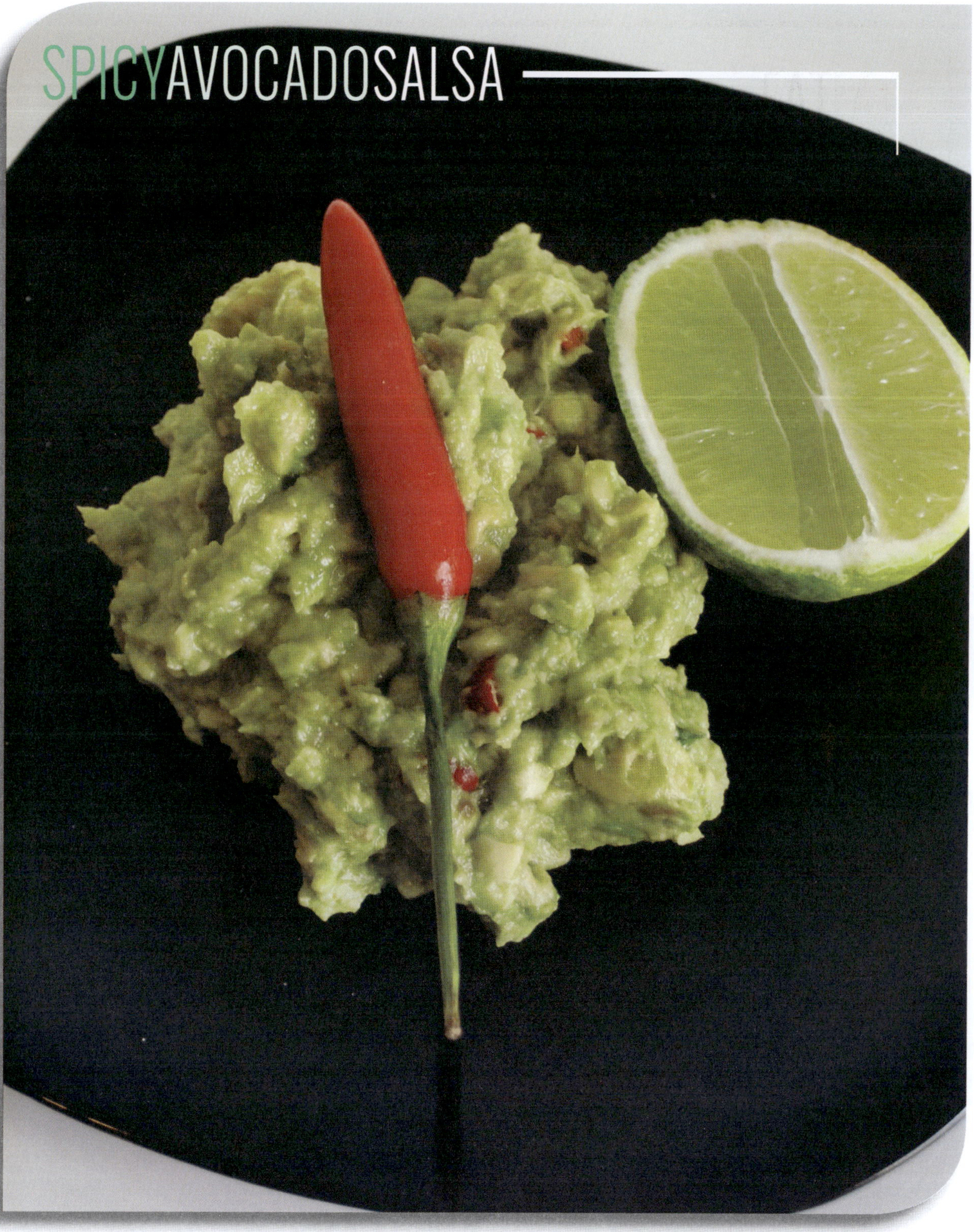

CREAMY TAHINI

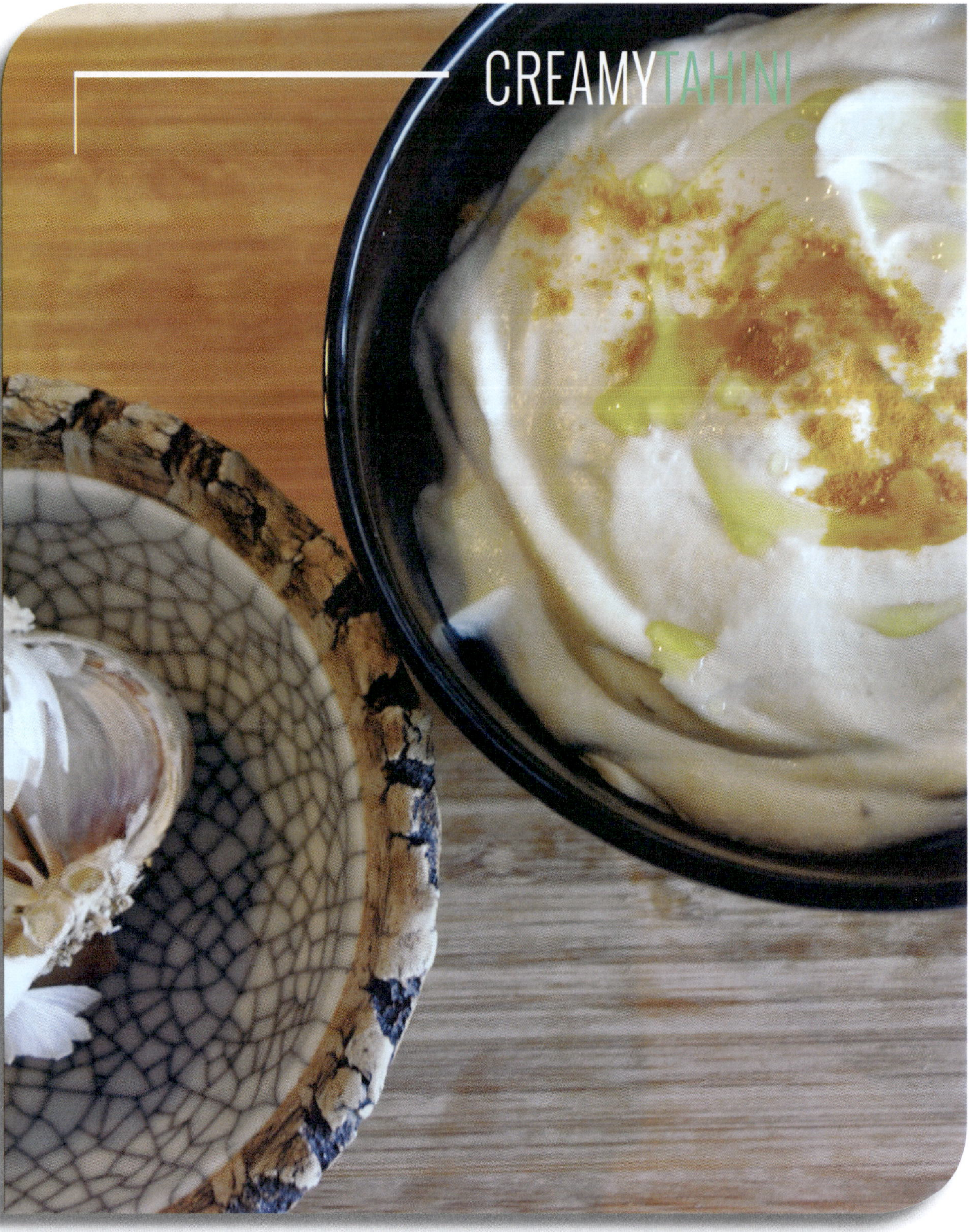

CREAMYTAHINI

Serves 6

Ingredients

1 jar unhulled tahini
Sea salt
1 large clove of garlic
1 whole lemon, juiced
Turmeric to garnish

Method

Empty the whole jar of tahini into a food processor. Fill the jar with water, filtered if you have it and add to food processor with crushed garlic clove and blend until it changes to a whiter colour.

Then add salt and lemon juice and blend again.

Taste it to see if you need more salt or garlic, depending on your taste. Pour into a bowl and sprinkle with turmeric or paprika. To keep fresh and to add taste, you can add a virgin cold pressed olive oil on top.

SARDINECUPS

Serves 6

Ingredients

6 endive leaves (used as cups)
6 sardine fillets (fresh or jar)
1 red capsicum, finely chopped
2 spring onions finely chopped
Juice of one lemon
Parsley

Method

Combine sardines, capsicum, spring onions and lemon juice to make a mixture.

Spoon into endive cups.

Season and serve.

SARDINE CUPS

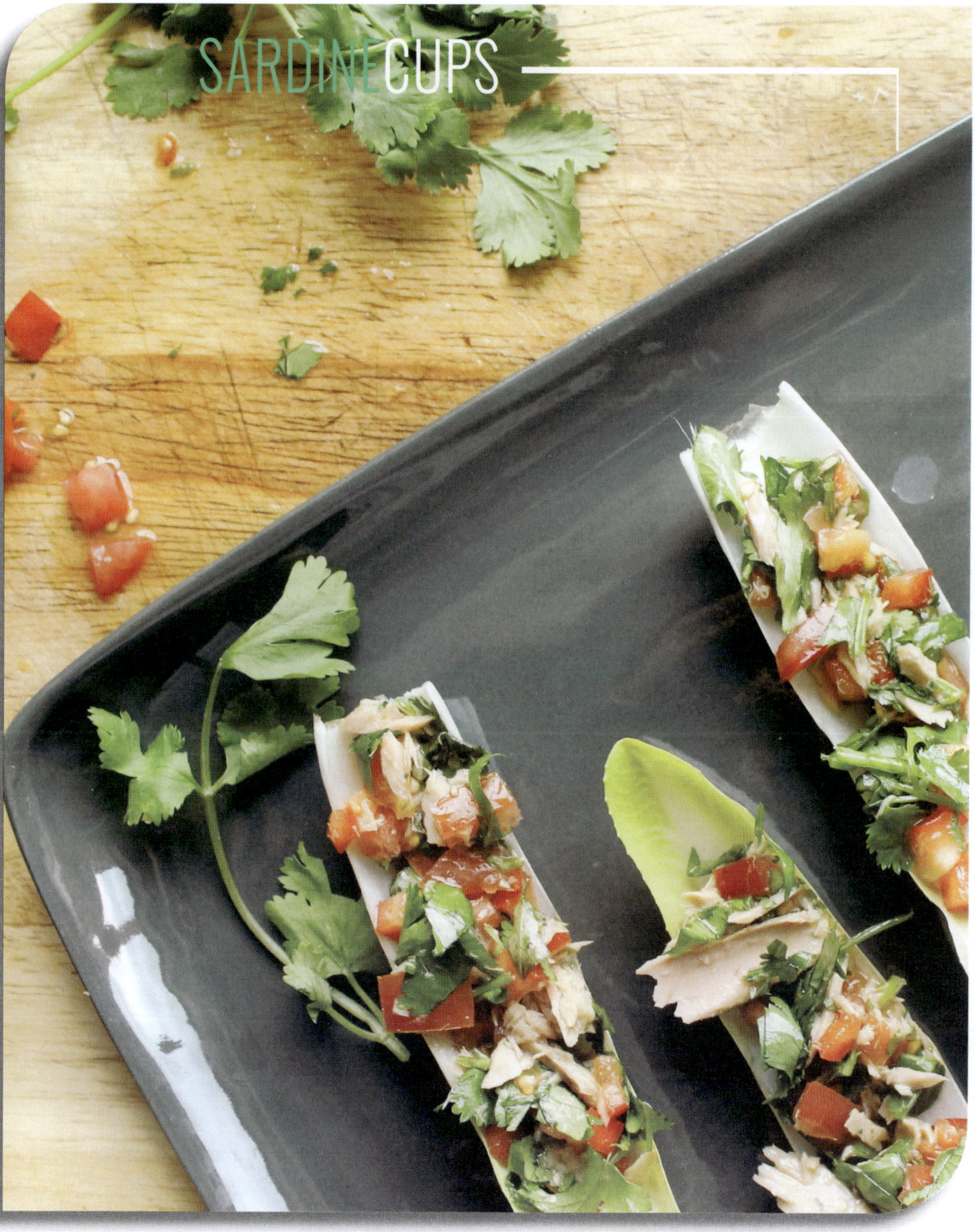

RADISH TZATZIKI

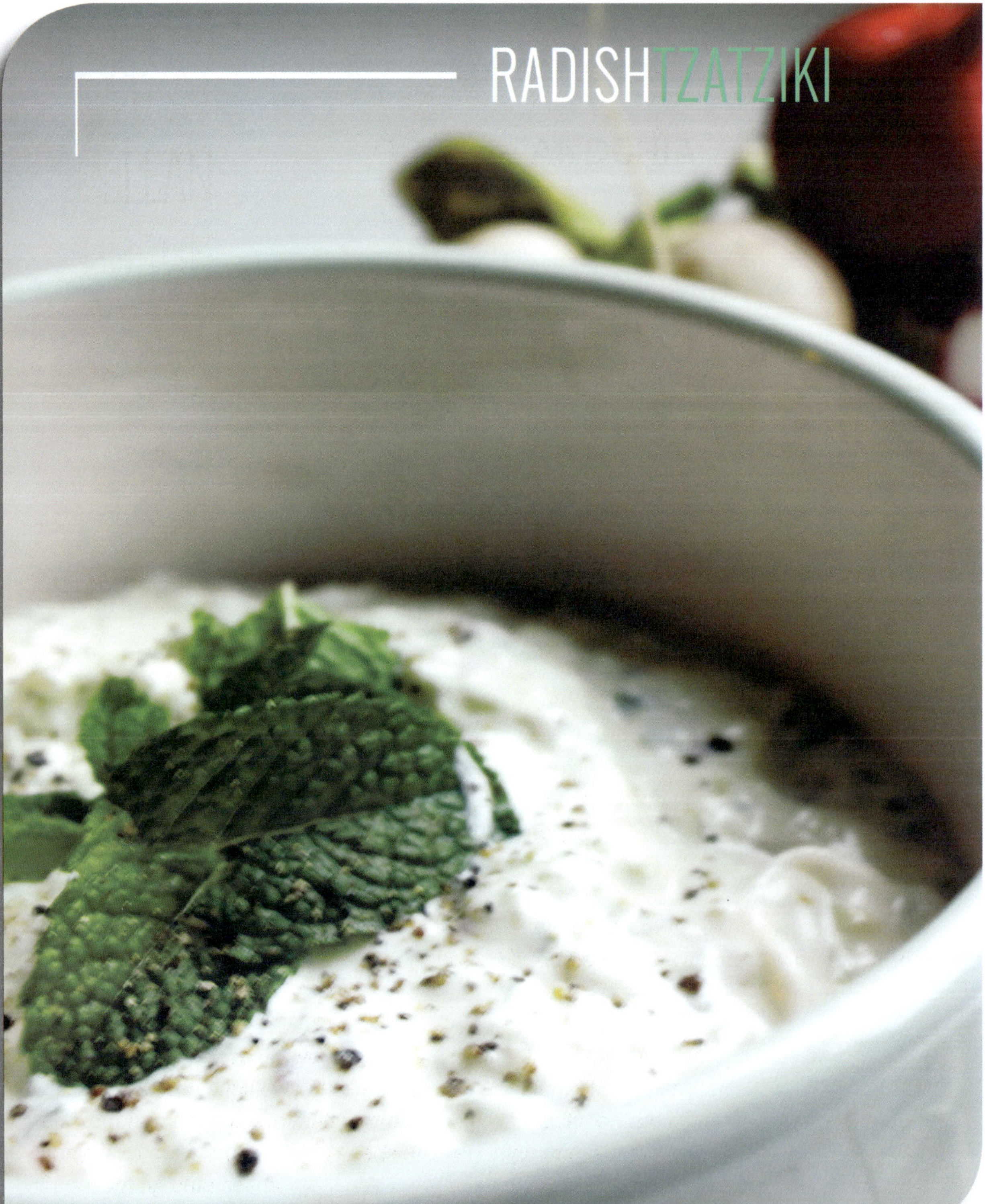

RADISHTZATZIKI

Ingredients

200 – 300ml of natural Greek yoghurt

5 radishes, chopped into ¼

1 Lebanese cucumber, chopped

Juice of 1/2 a lemon

Rind of 1/2 lemon

3 tbls extra virgin olive oil

A generous pinch of salt

Mint to garnish

Method

In a food processor (or you could grate), combine the radish and cucumber and very roughly chop. Squeeze out any excess liquid.

Place in a bowl and add yoghurt. Combine. Add lemon juice and rind, oil and salt and stir well. If the mix is too runny, add a touch more yoghurt.

Garnish with mint and cracked pepper – serve with veggie sticks (carrot, celery, snow peas etc)

ORANGE AND CHIA SEED CAKE

Serves 12

Ingredients

2 oranges – tops removed / cut and scored with a cross about 3cm deep
6 organic free-range eggs
250g xylitol
250g almond meal
3 tsp baking powder
2 tbls soaked chia seeds

Method

Place the prepared oranges in boiling water and simmer for 50 minutes. Remove from the water and purée the whole orange, including peel in a food processor, until smooth.

Preheat the oven to 160 °C. In a large mixing bowl, mix the eggs and xylitol until light and fluffy. Add the almond meal and baking powder. Mix until combined. Stir in the orange purée and soaked chia seeds. Pour the mixture into a 22cm cake tin lined with greaseproof baking paper. Do not use foil.

Bake in the oven for 40 minutes or until firm but still moist. It may need to cook for up to 50 minutes. Leave to cool in the tin for about 5 minutes then turn onto a wire rack and cool there.

Note: This cake is a really wet cake and can stay fresh for a few days. It can be served warm with sheep's milk yoghurt dolloped on the side. The almond meal provides a gluten-free treat and once again high in protein. This is a twist on the traditional orange and poppy seed cake, but the chia seeds are very high in essential fatty acids. It's a great way of consuming chia seeds.

ORANGE AND CHIA SEED CAKE

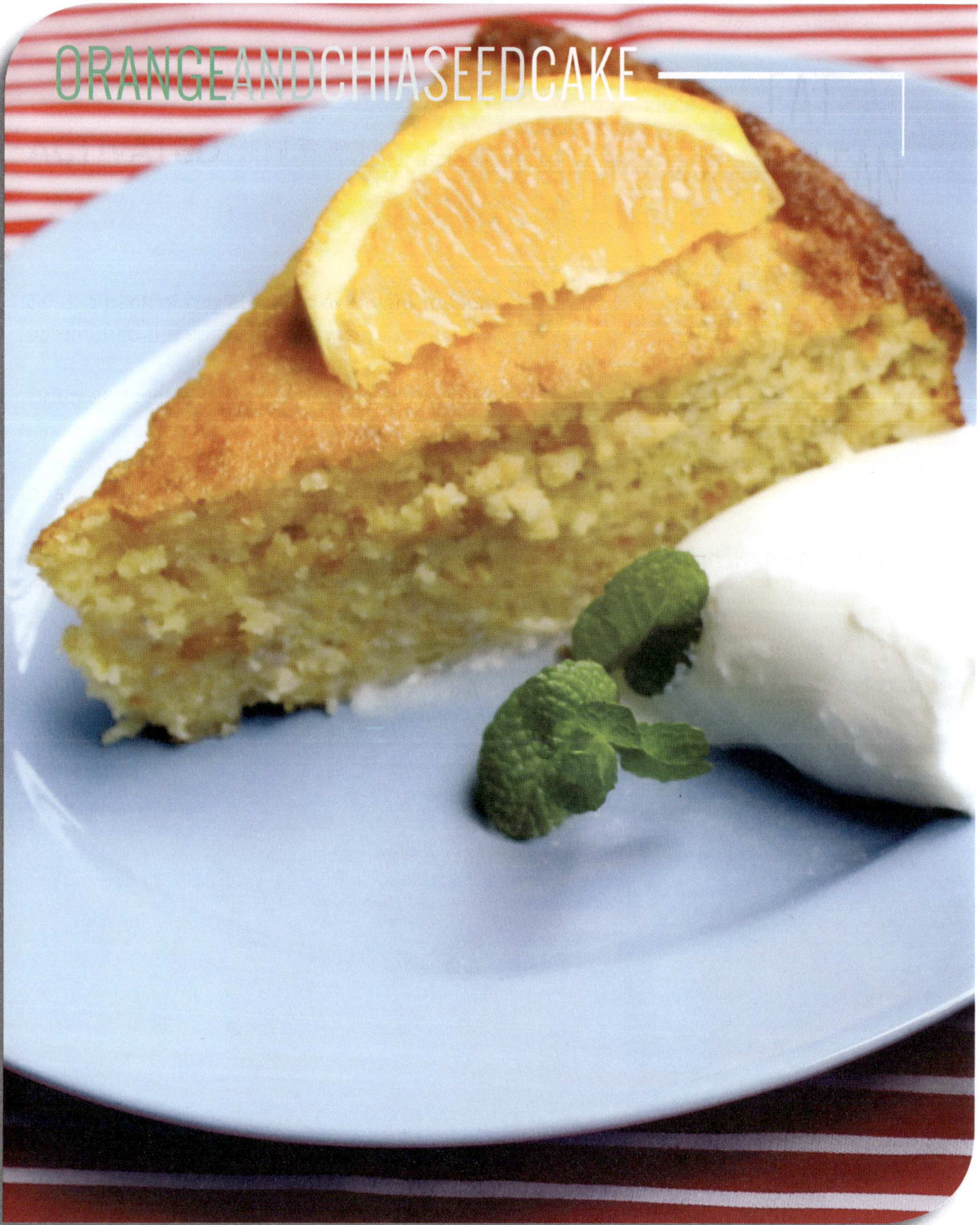

ACTIVATED NUTS

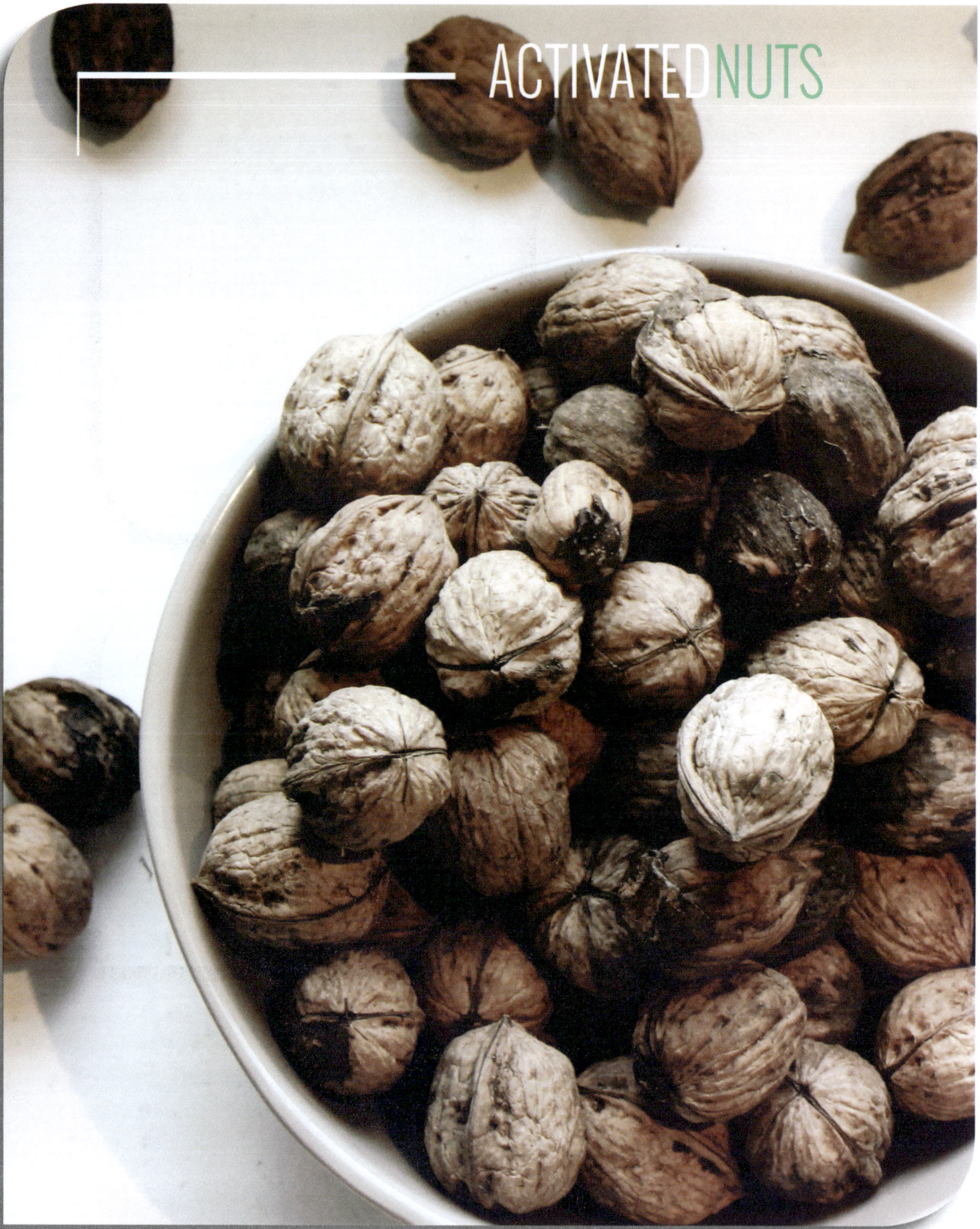

ACTIVATED**NUTS**

Soak a pack of raw almonds overnight to 'activate' and commence the sprouting process.

Drain and place on an oven tray ready to bake.

Place in an oven on the lowest heat (around 60°C) and cook for at least 12 hours (yes, you heard us - 12 hours!)

Enjoy as a snack whenever, add to salads, muffins - any way you can get them in. Even munch on these for a 4pm pick me up. Store in a glass jar.

Always, always soak your nuts and rice overnight. It makes them easy to digest not to mention rids them of toxic phytic acid, which can be found in the skin of the nut/rice and is bad news for your body.

SALADS

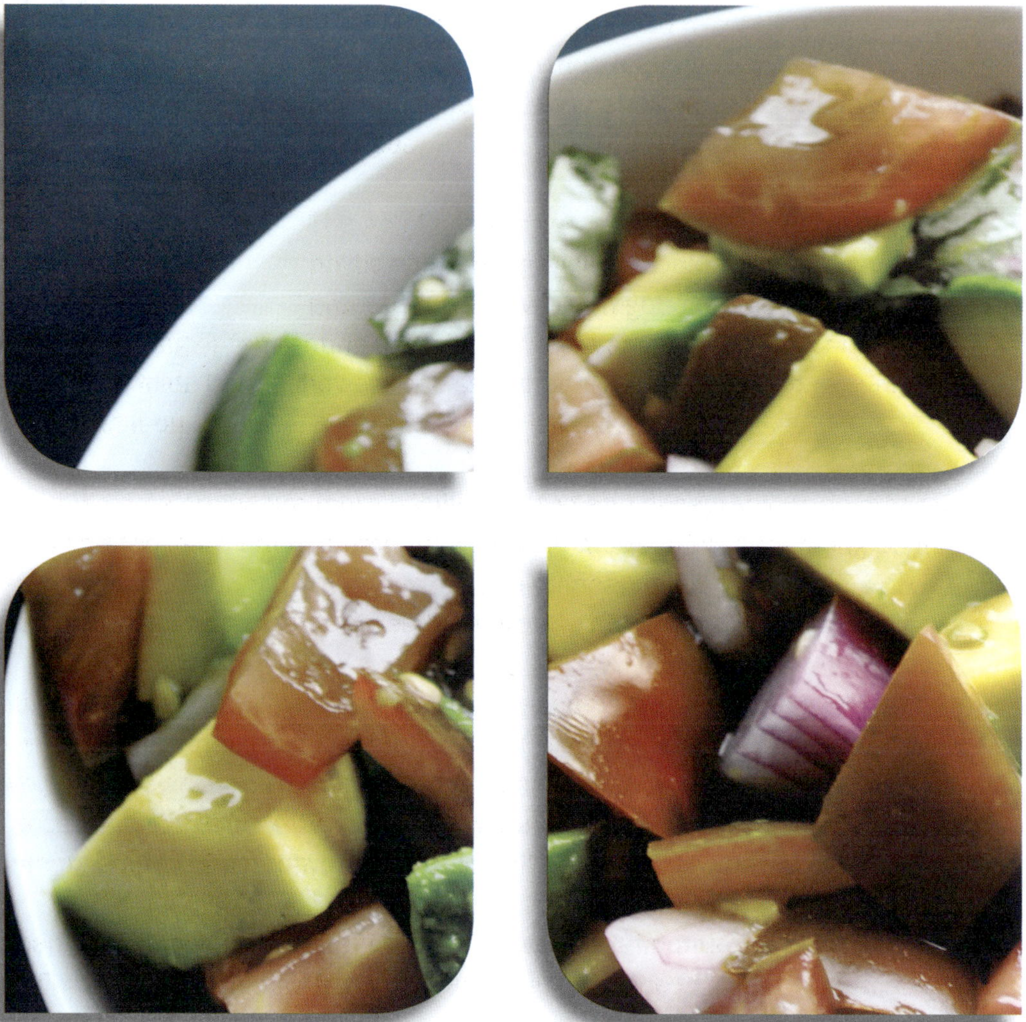

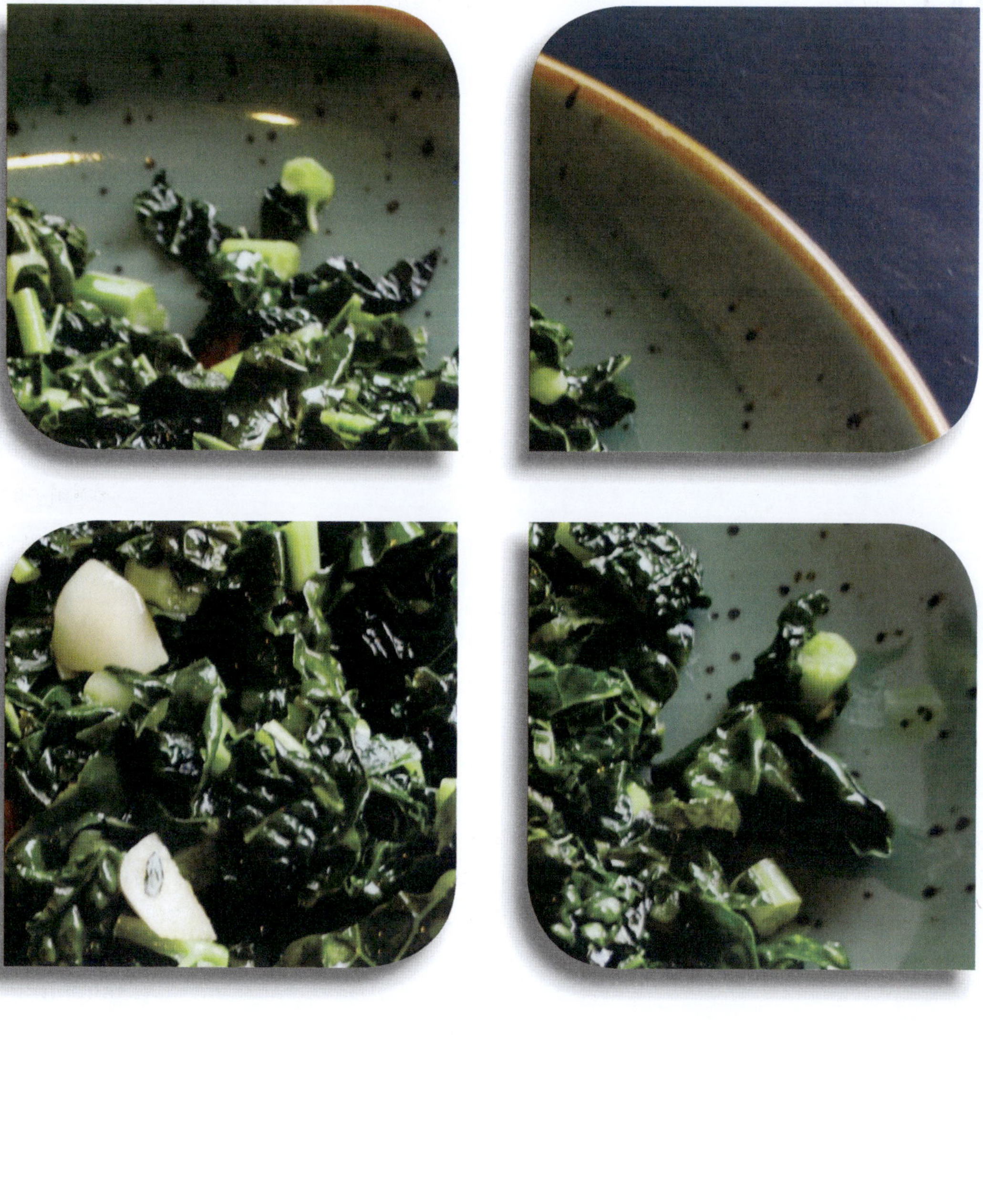

SALADS

SMOKED SALMON SALAD

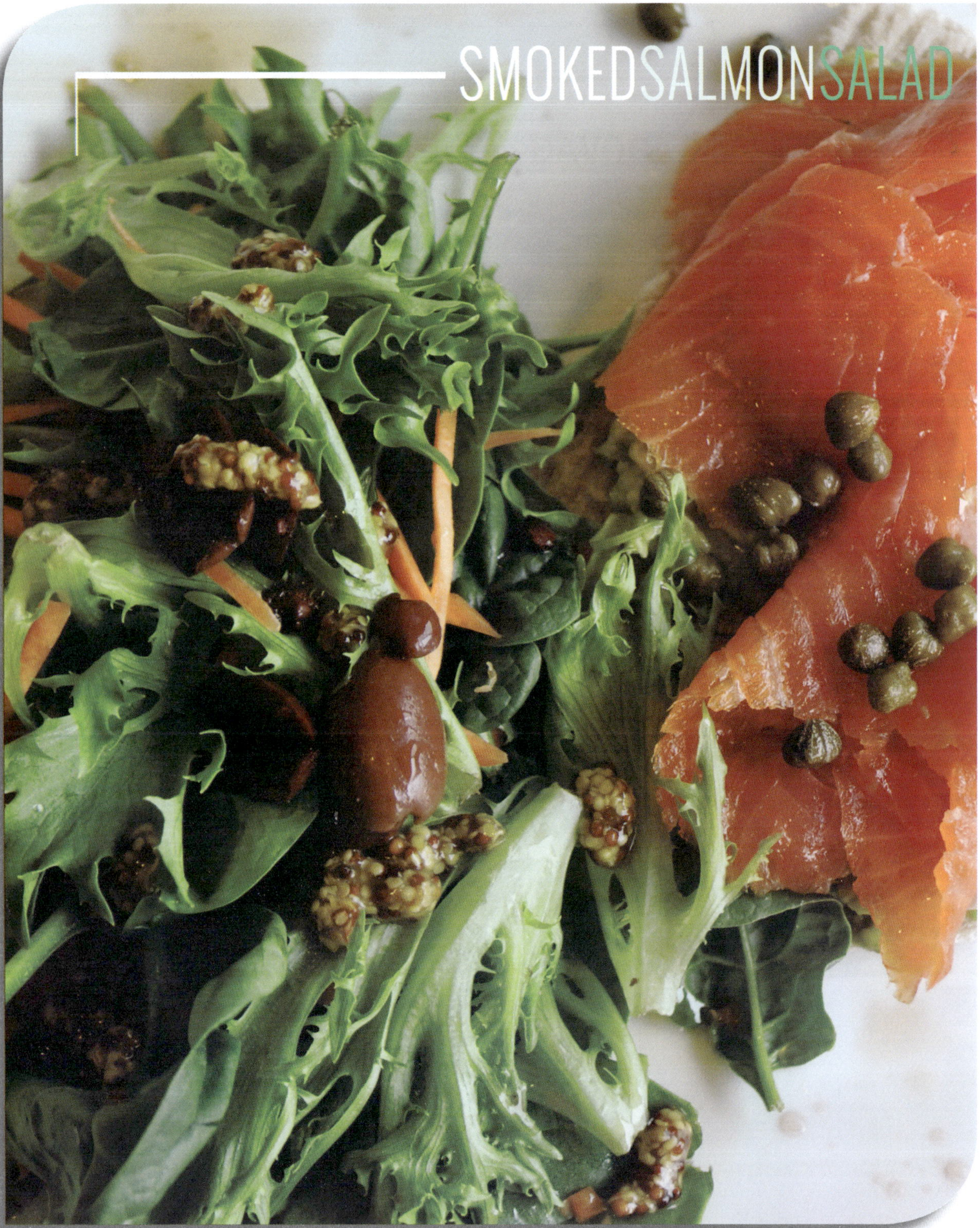

SMOKEDSALMONSALAD

Serves 1

Ingredients

200g smoked salmon

2 rye or gluten and wheat free rice crackers

Seeded mustard

A handful of mixed green lettuce and grated carrot

Lemon juice

Capers

Cracked black pepper

Olives

¼ avocado

Method

Scoop out the avocado onto the crackers and top with salmon and capers. Throw lettuce and grated carrot together, with olives and capers. To make dressing, mix the juice of a lemon and seeded mustard with sea salt and pepper and drizzle over the salad.

Eat immediately.

BASILANDAVOCADOSALAD

Serves 4

Ingredients

2 ripe avocados
Sea salt
2 cucumbers
6 large organic tomatoes or 14 cherry tomatoes
1 purple onion
A bunch of fresh basil
Lemon
Cracked black pepper

Method

Chop all ingredients into squares. Tear basil leaves and mix all together, squeeze the whole juice of a lemon, add a third of a cup of avocado oil and salt and pepper to taste.

Serve with any main meal or any protein.

BASIL AND AVOCADO SALAD

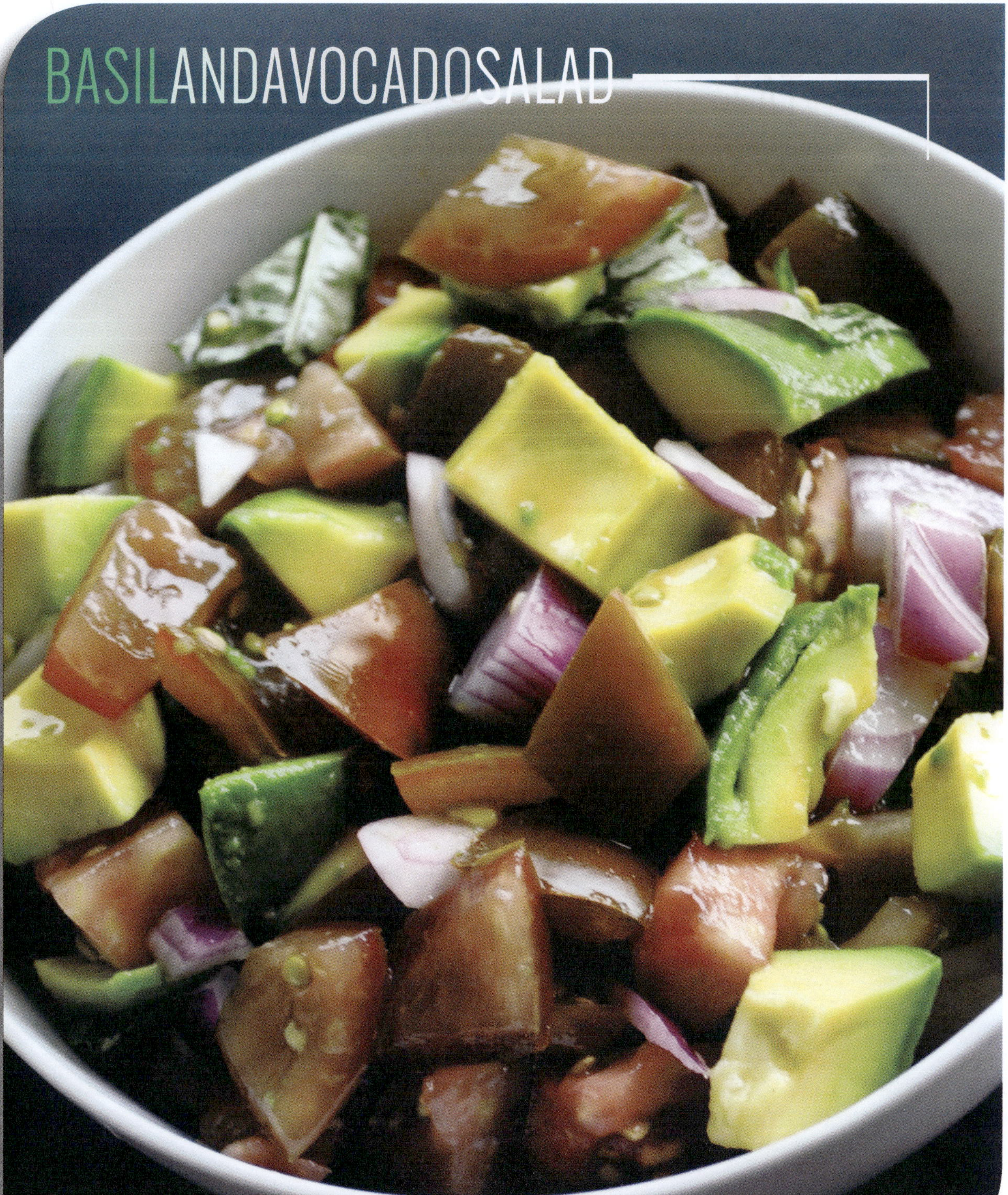

ISRAELI CABBAGE SALAD

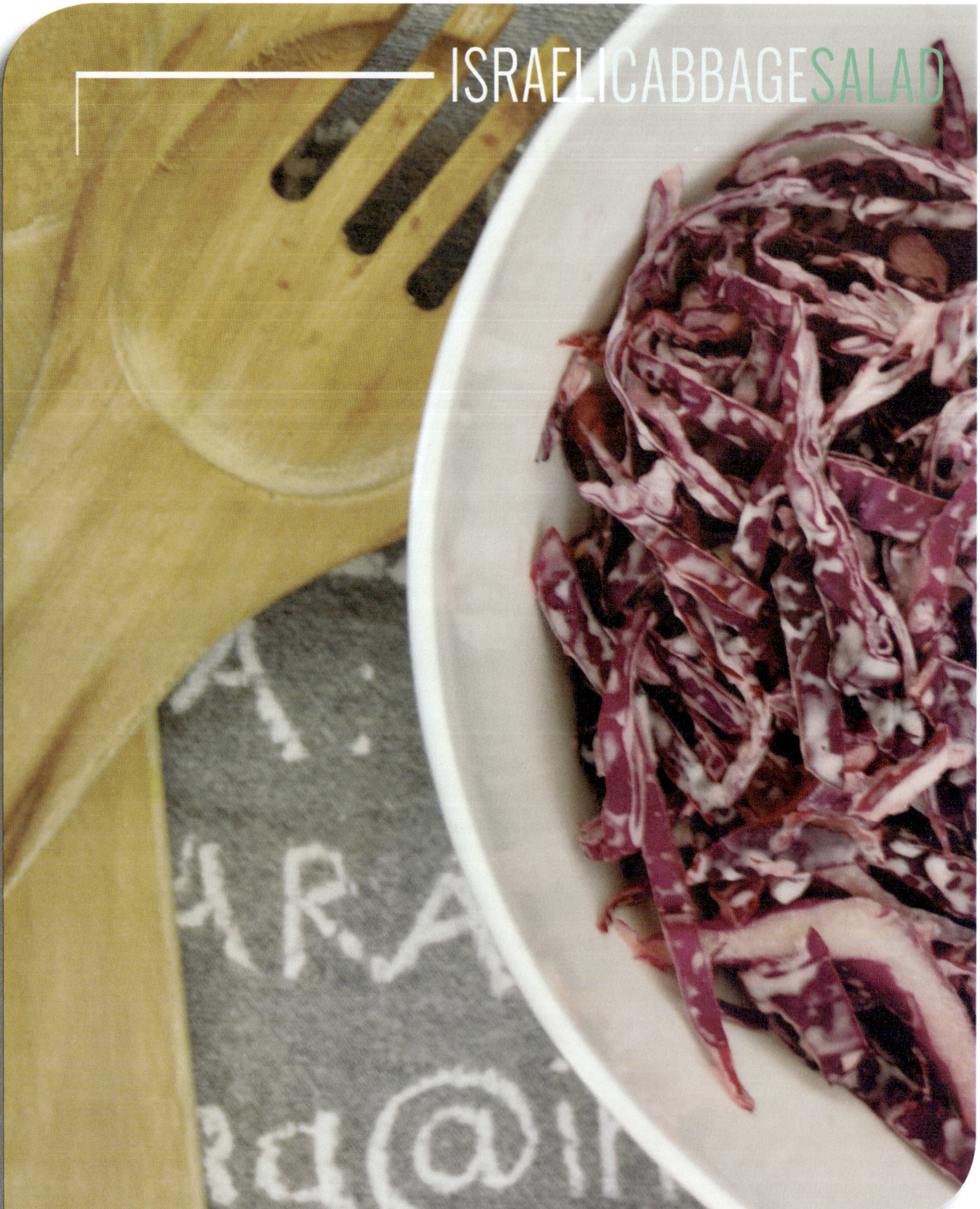

ISRAELICABBAGESALAD

Serves 4

Ingredients

Half a large purple cabbage

3 tbls whole egg or soy mayonnaise (sugar free)

2 gloves crushed garlic

1 fresh lemon (juiced)

Sea salt

Method

Finely cut the cabbage and place in a bowl. Add all other ingredients and stir. It tastes better when you let it sit in the fridge for about half an hour, but served right away, it's also very tasty!

WARMKALESALAD

Serves 4

Ingredients

1 bunch of kale
Sea salt
2 large cloves of garlic
Fresh red chilli
2 tbls organic cold pressed coconut oil

Method

Chop kale into fine strips. Heat pan with 2 tbls organic cold pressed coconut oil. Smash and peel the garlic cloves and add to the oil, lightly cook then add the kale and chopped chilli. Add salt to taste and cook until kale softens a little.

Serve and eat warm immediately.

WARM KALE SALAD

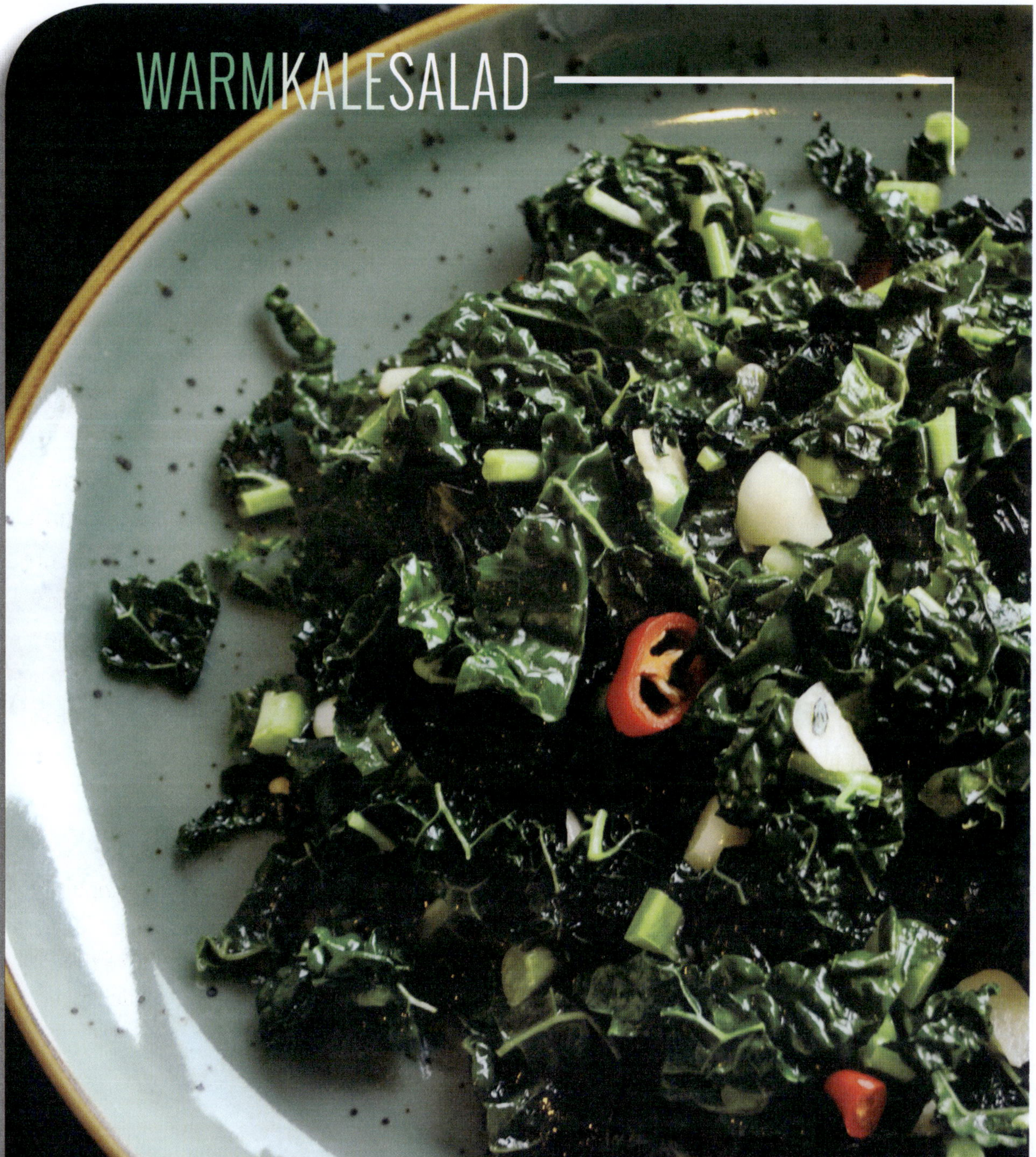

MUSHROOM SALAD

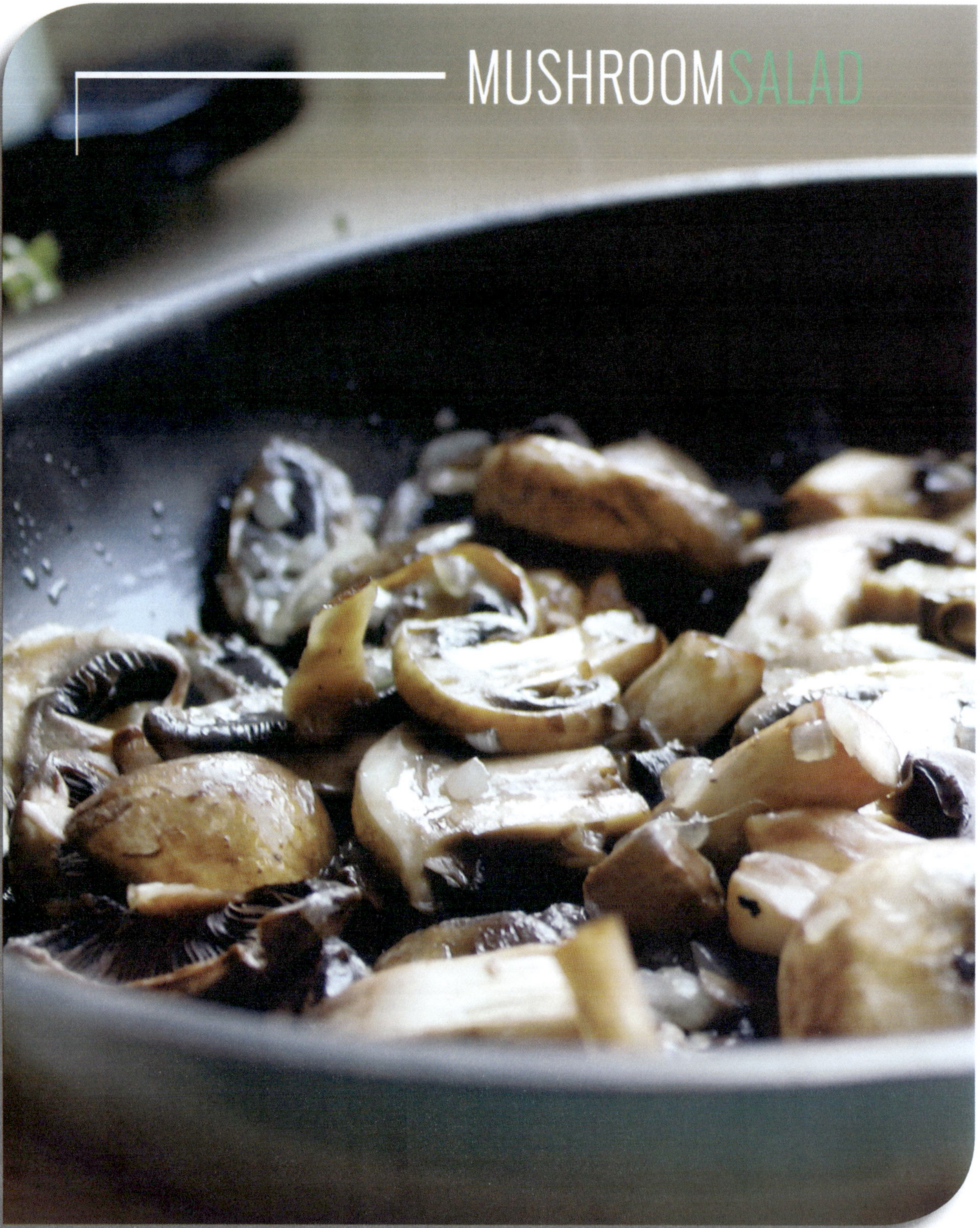

MUSHROOMSALAD

Serves 4

Ingredients

1 onion

500g mushrooms of your choice – you might like to mix several varieties

Coconut oil to shallow fry

Apple cider vinegar

Chilli to serve

Method

Dice onion.

Add a tablespoon of coconut oil to a fry pan. Add onion and mushrooms. Allow to cook through.

Remove from head and add to a bowl. Stir through a splash of apple cider vinegar and chilli to garnish.

IMMUNEBOOSTINGORANGE ANDFENNELSALAD

Serves 2

Ingredients

2 large fennels
2 oranges
Half a purple onion
Olive oil - 3 tbls
Peruvian salt from Powersuperfoods

Method

Cut orange and fennel pieces into bite size squares. Cut onion into smaller chunks.

Mix in a bowl with olive oil and two good pinches of salt.

Eat straight away!

ORANGE AND FENNEL SALAD

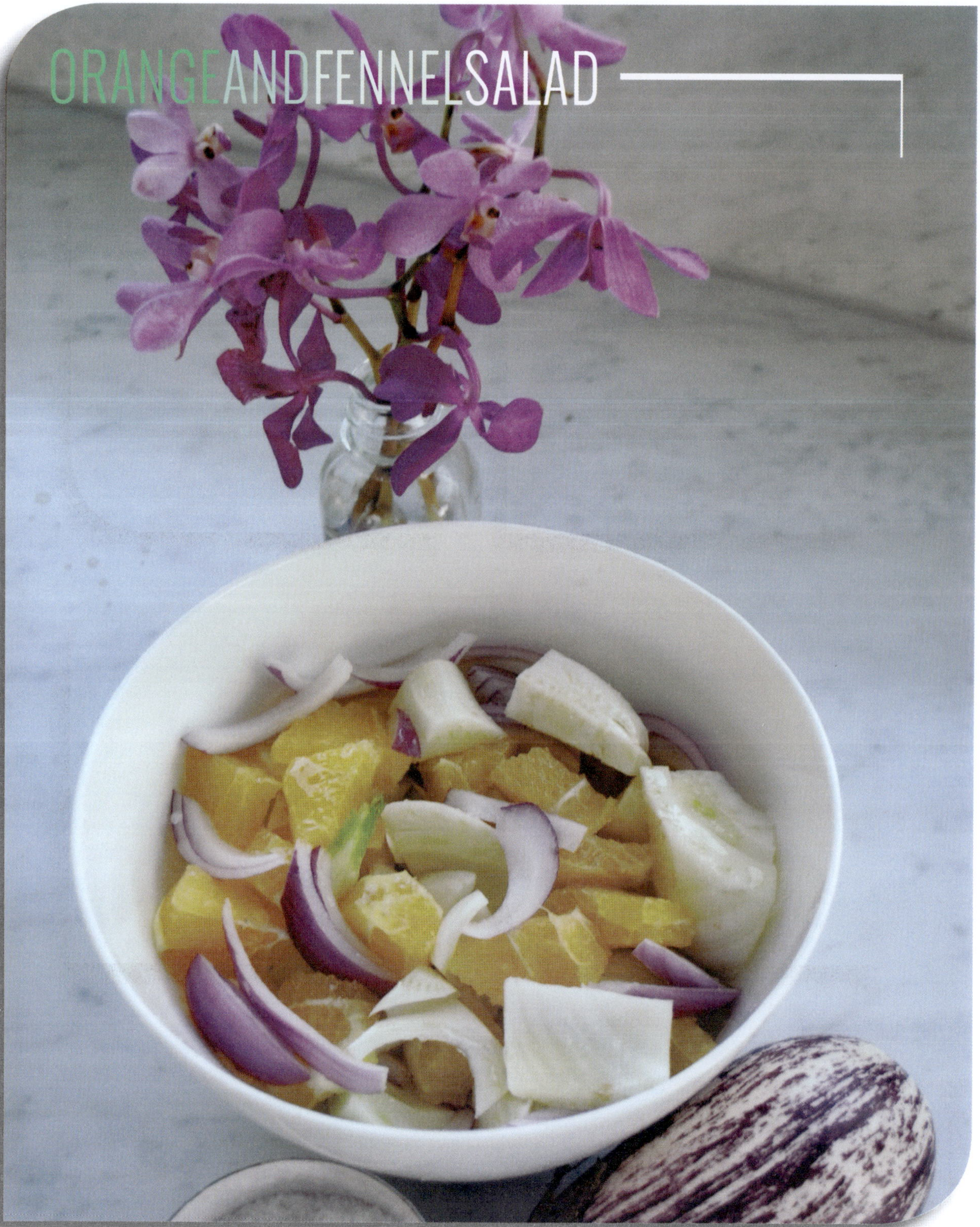

SOUPS

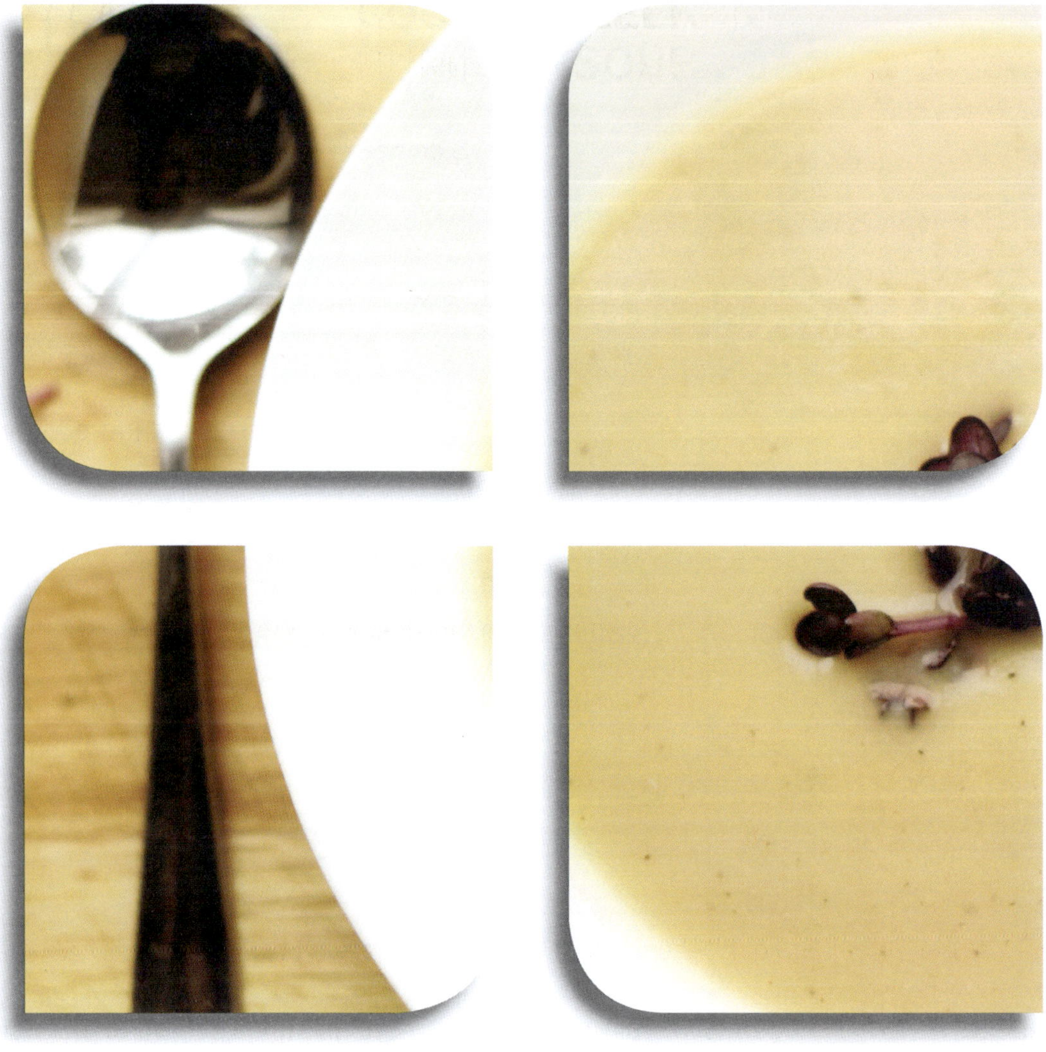

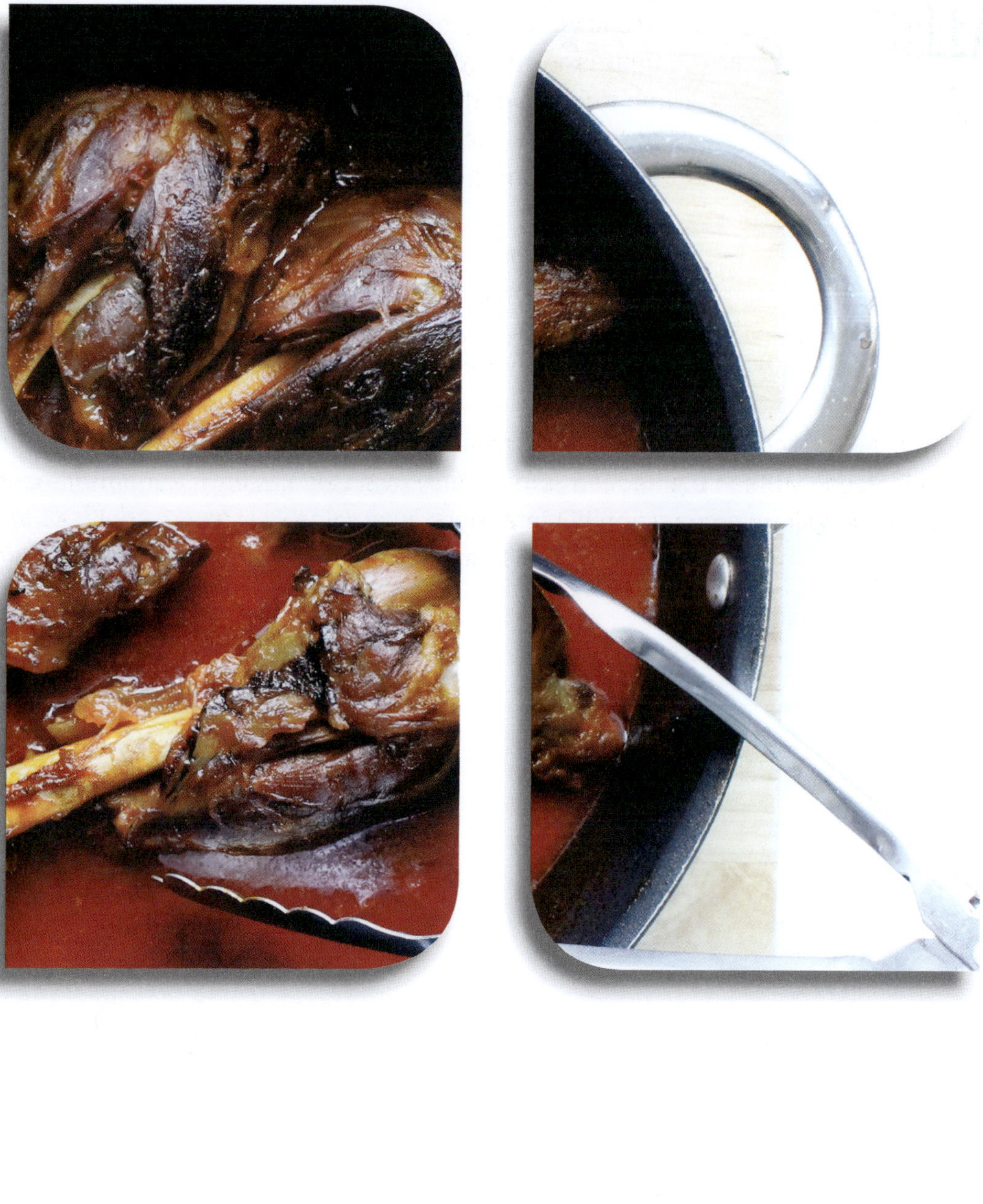

SOUPS

COCONUT, LEEK AND PUMPKIN SOUP

Serves 6

Ingredients

1 butternut pumpkin
Sea salt
2 large sweet potatoes
2 brown onions
1 leek
2 organic non GMO, no additives vegetable stock cubes
Cracked black pepper
1 litre water
4 tbls organic cold pressed coconut oil
1 bunch of fresh coriander

Method

Peel and cut the pumpkin and sweet potato into large cubes. Chop onion and leeks.

Fry onion and leeks in a soup pot or pressure cooker with coconut oil. Add water, pumpkin, sweet potato, stock cubes, coriander and put on to boil. Once boiled, let it simmer for 15-20 mins until vegetables are soft.

Blend with a blender or hand held blender. Serve with a dollop of coconut oil and a sprig of coriander for garnish.

COCONUT LEEK AND PUMPKIN SOUP

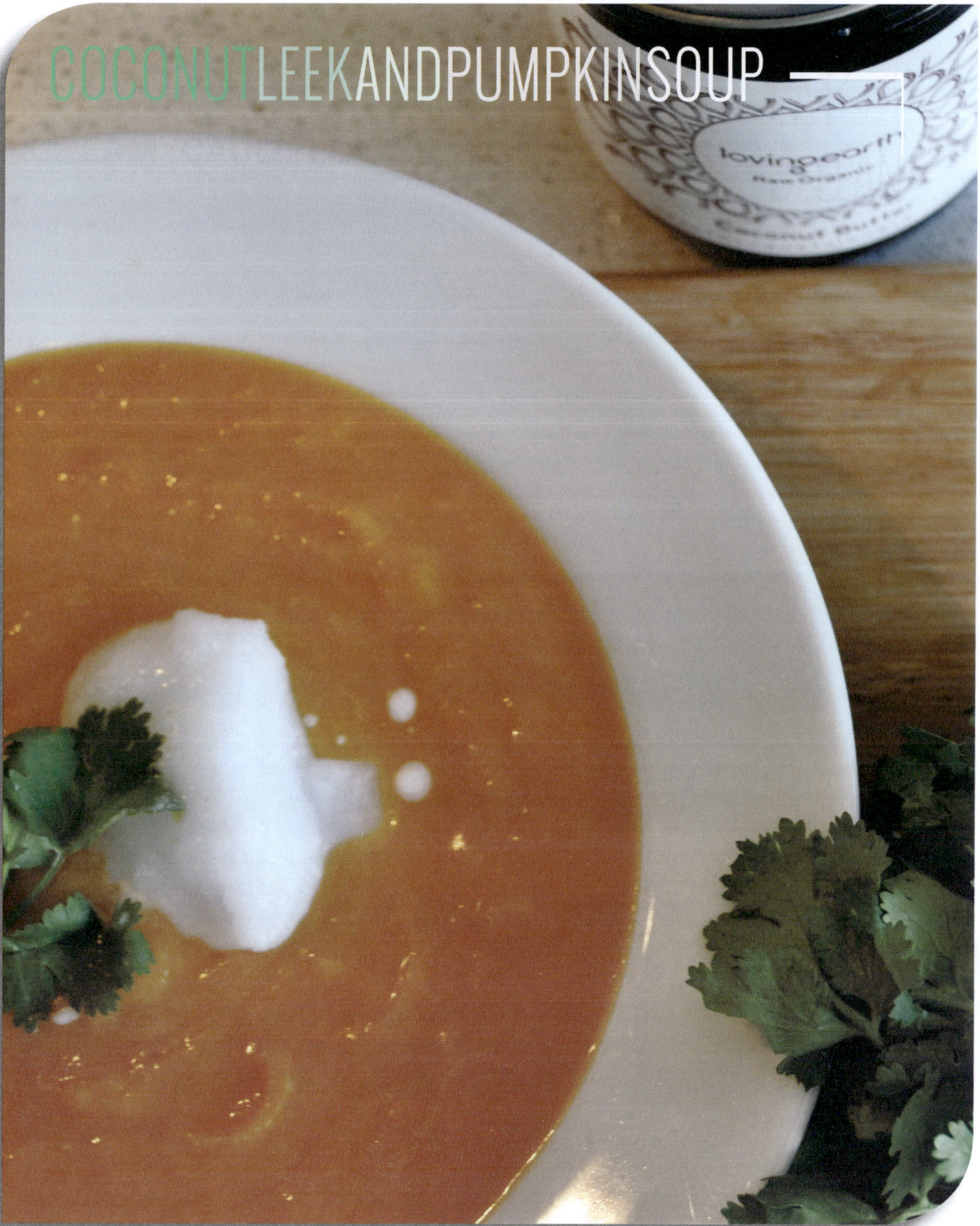

CREAMY CAULIFLOWER SOUP

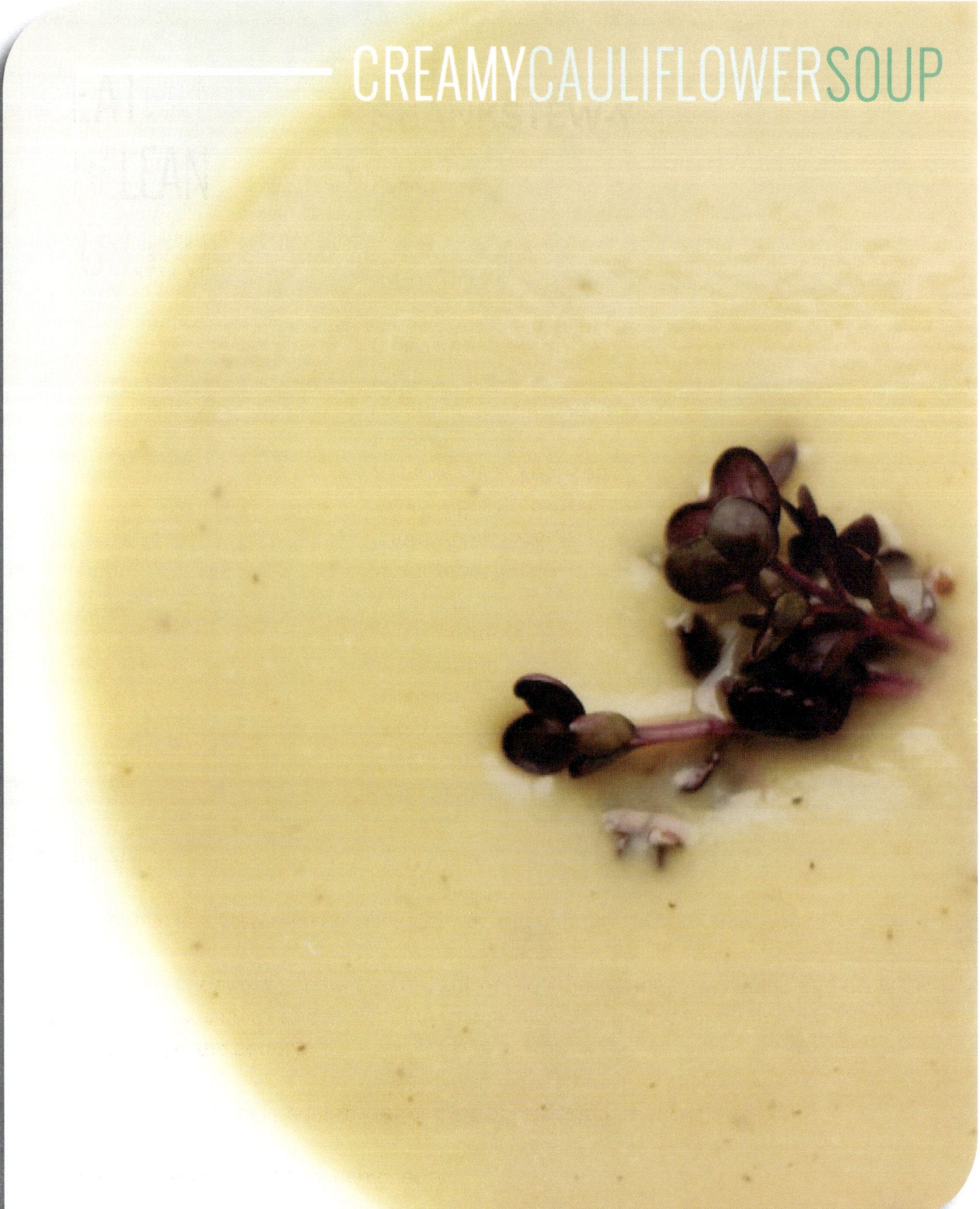

CREAMYCAULIFLOWERSOUP

Serves 6

Ingredients

1/3 cup of coconut oil
1 medium sized cauliflower broken into florets
2 medium sizes onions, roughly chopped
3 garlic cloves, roughly chopped
5 cups of stock
1 cup of almond milk

Method

Heat oil in a large pot, adding onion and garlic. Allow to cook for a few minutes until they start to become clear.

Add cauliflower and allow it to begin to brown.

Cover with stock and allow it to come to the boil. Reduce heat and cook for 30 minutes (the longer the better) until the cauliflower is soft and breaks up easily.

Run Wizz Stick mixer or put into the blender until there are no lumps and the soup is a very smooth consistency.

Place back onto the heat and add almond milk.
Serve with crusty bread and garnish with parsley and pepper.

AR-MAZING! It doesn't even taste like cauliflower soup! So delicious.

SHANKSTEW-YSOUP

Serves 4-6

Ingredients

6 lamb shanks
2 tbls coconut oil
2 onions roughly chopped
1 carrot chopped
1 celery stick, chopped
1 sweet potato chopped
1 tomato chopped
½ a lemon, juiced
2 tsp salt
½ tsp turmeric
½ tsp cumin
½ tsp paprika
½ tsp cinnamon
4 cups of stock
Parmesan to garnish

Method

Brown shanks in a very large pot. Once brown add onions and cook until soft.

Add carrot, celery, sweet potato, tomato, spices, seasoning and lemon juice and allow to slightly brown. Add stock and allow bring to boil. Allow to simmer for a minimum of one hour (the longer the better).

Remove shanks and pull meat away from the bone. Return meat to the pot.

Serve with a sprinkle of parmesan cheese.

SHANK STEWY SOUP

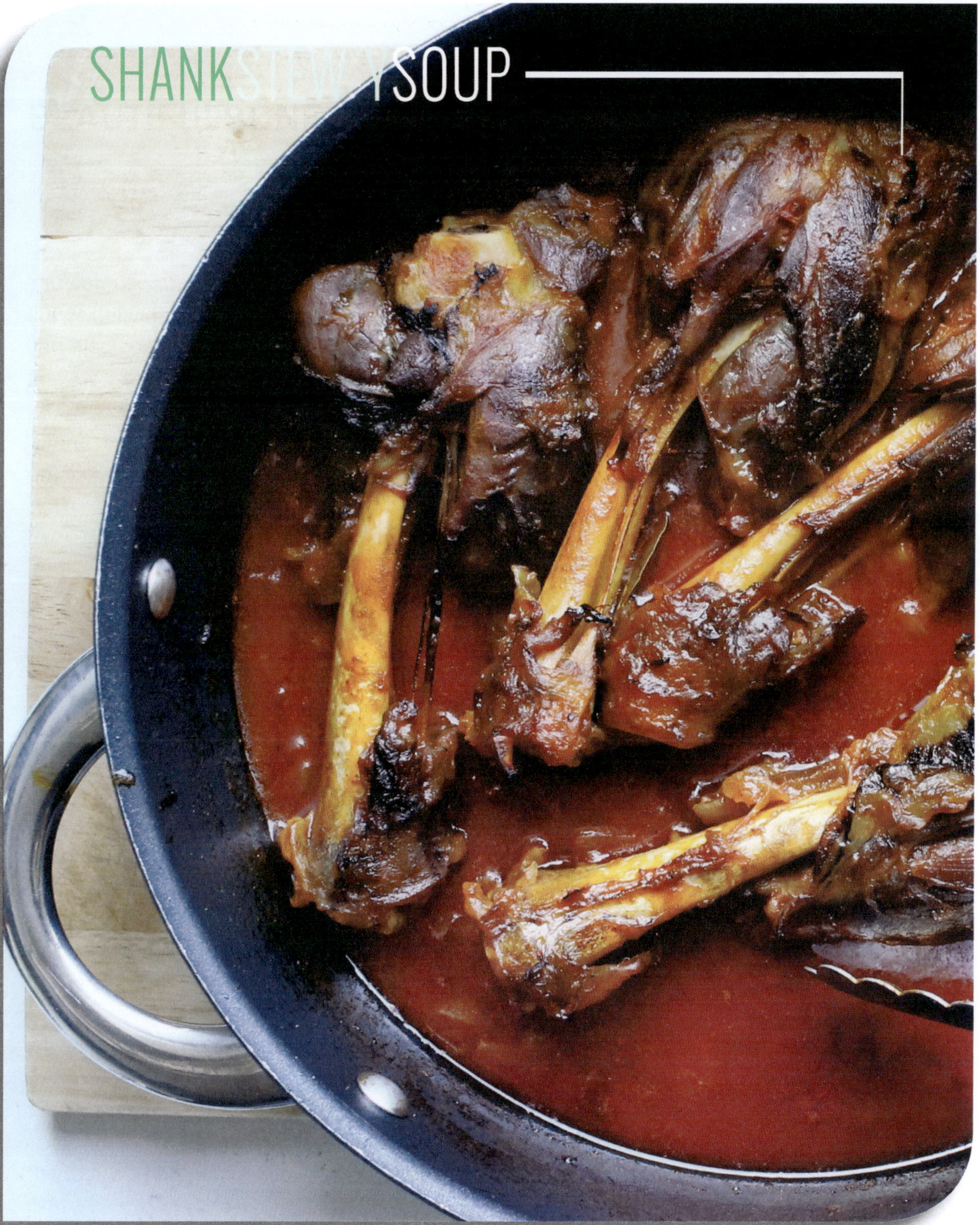

BEAUTIFUL BONE BROTH

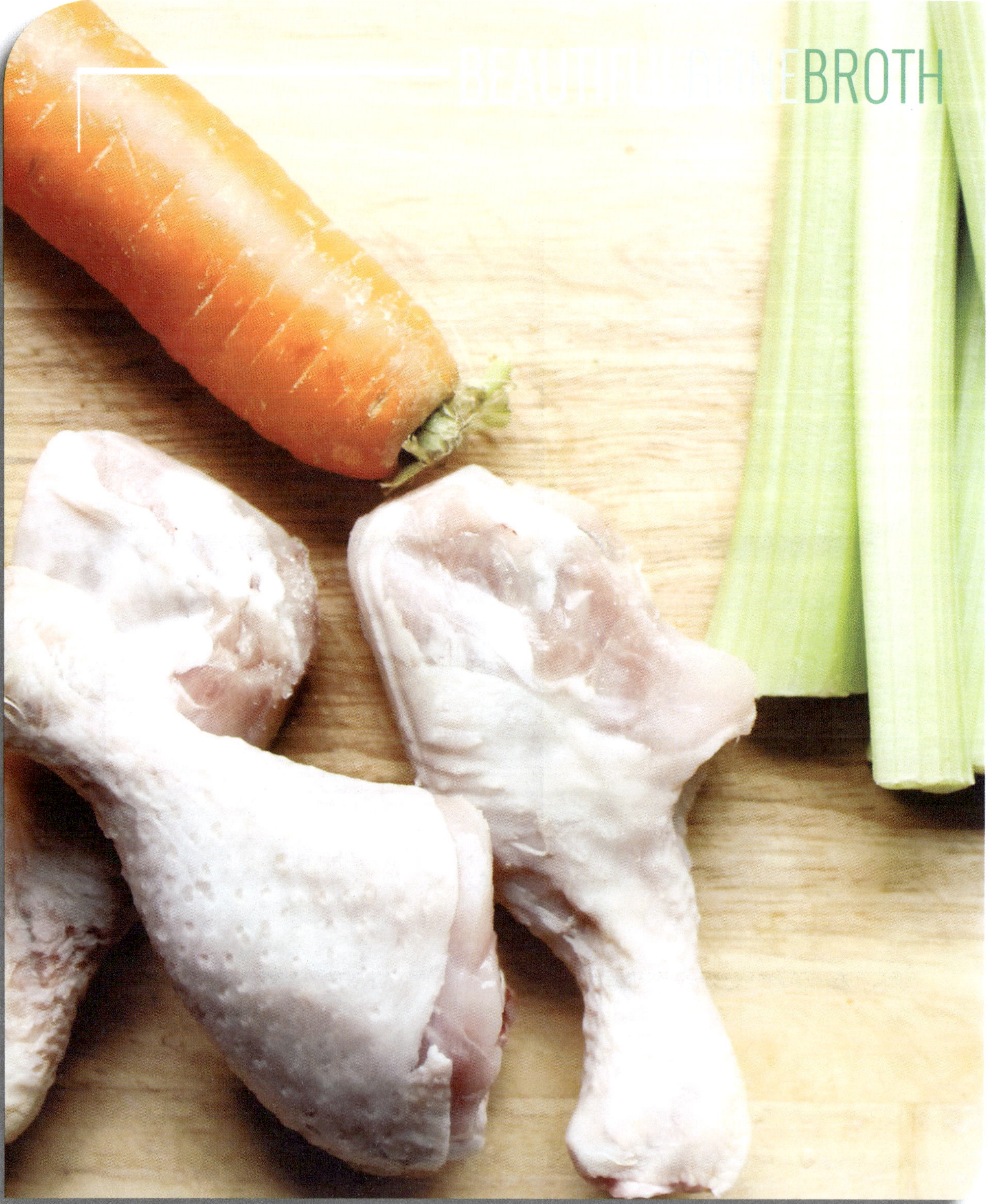

BEAUTIFULBONEBROTH

Makes 3 litres

You can use any bones you like to make this broth. It is super delicious and excellent to balance hormones. You can also cook up a big batch of this and freeze it to use in soups and stews as stock.

1 large chicken or 2 kg of bones (beef, ribs, neck bones – whatever you can get your hands on)

Ingredients

3 litres of cold water
½ cup of vinegar
3 carrots chopped
3 celery sticks chopped
Thyme and parsley tied together to easily remove once cooked
Pepper and salt

Method

Place bones, water and vinegar in a large pot and allow to sit.

If you have some bones with a lot of meat you might like to roast them before adding them to the pot. This helps bring out flavour. If you have a whole chicken, just add it.

Add carrot and celery to the pot – ensure there is enough water to cover.

Place on stove. The longer this simmers, the better to bring out the nutrients – some will cook this up to 72 hours! We suggest you simmer for as long as possible (5ish hours). In the last 30 minutes of cooking, add herbs and seasoning.

FISHANDMEAT

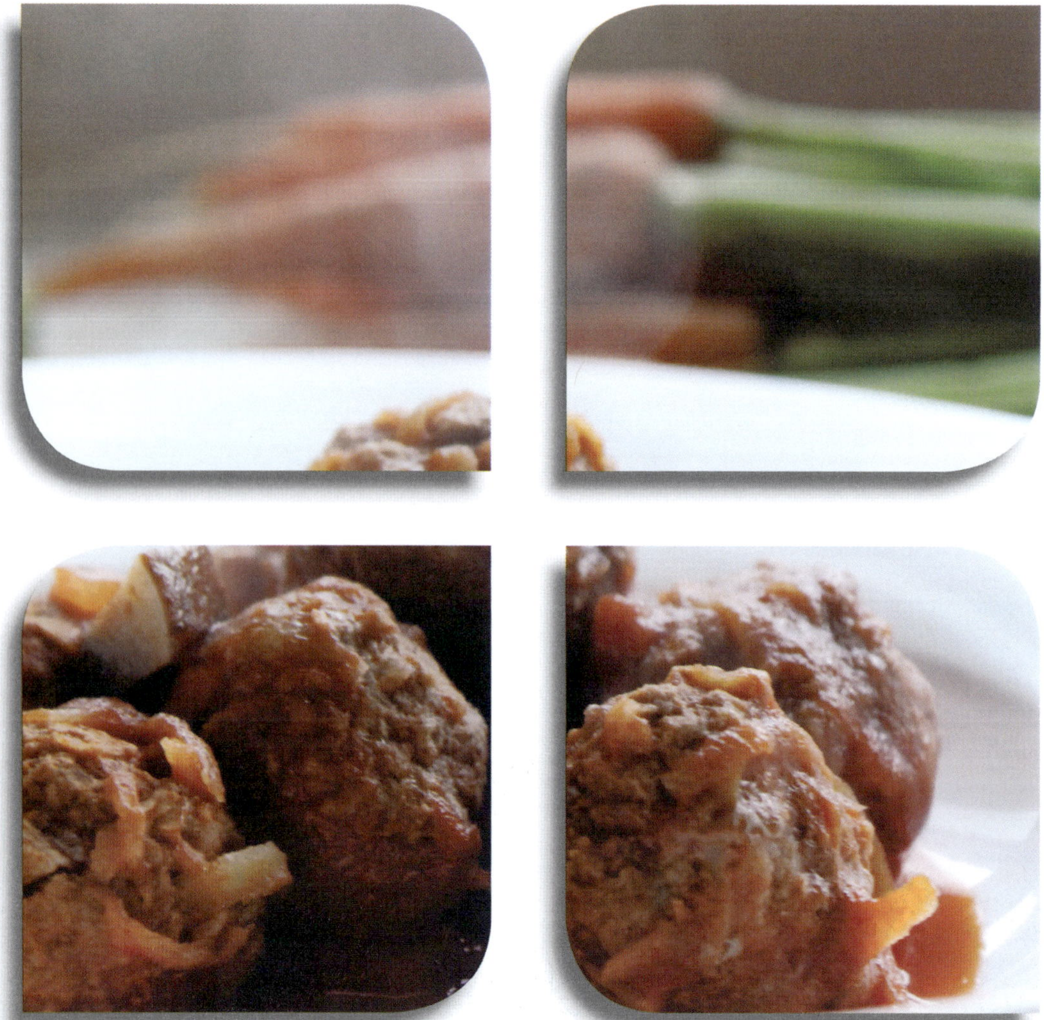

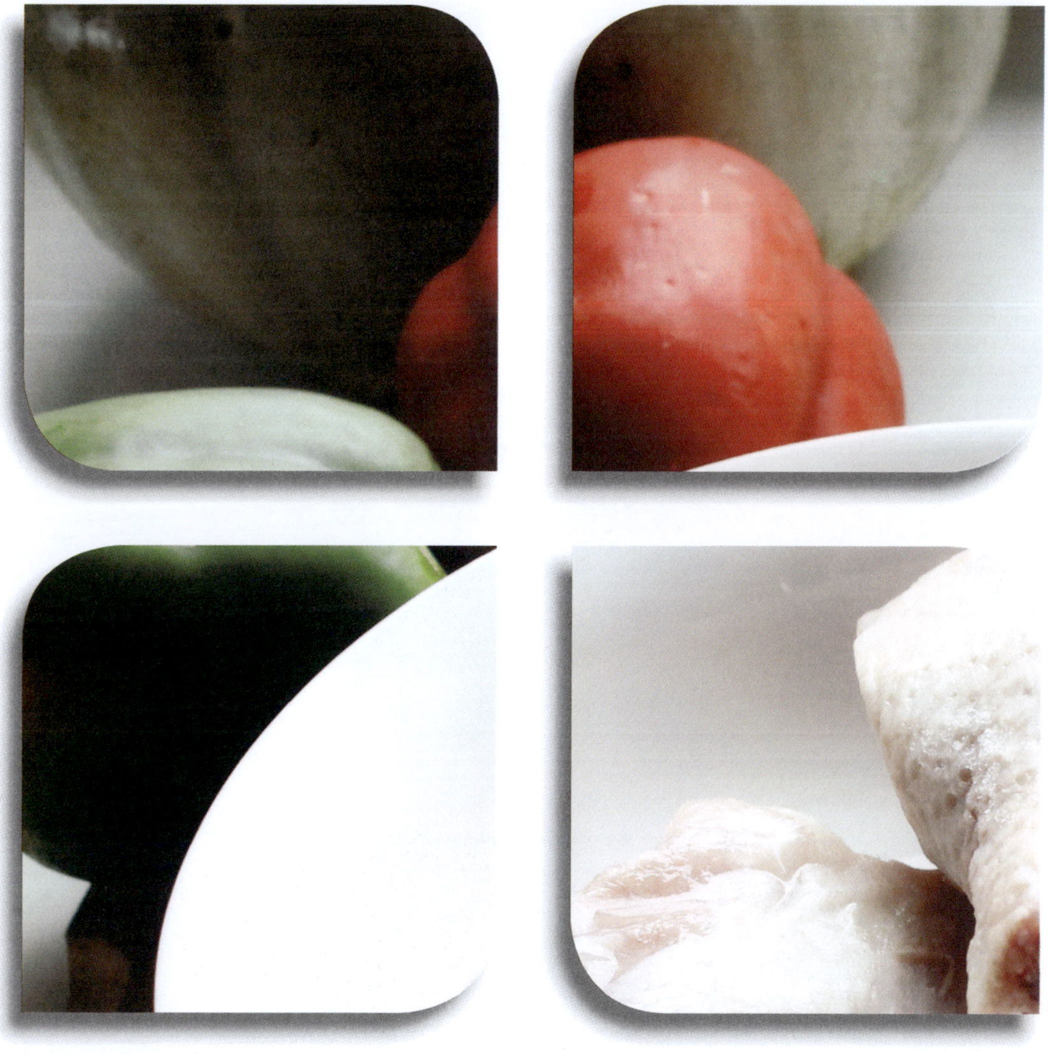

FISHANDMEAT

BRAZILIANSTYLEFISHWITH COCONUTMILK

Serves 3

Ingredients

1 large skinned Barramundi fillet or another white fleshy fish without bones (500g)
1 container of coconut milk or coconut cream
2 tbls of coconut oil
4 cloves of whole garlic pieces
1 brown onion
3 coloured capsicums, green, yellow and red
Fresh chilli (optional)
3 fresh tomatoes
Bunch of fresh coriander

Method

Peel and chop the onion in a fry pan with the coconut oil to brown. Add sliced capsicums, diced tomato and whole chilli. Leave the seeds in, but only remove the top. Cook for a few minutes. Move these ingredients to the side of the pan and sear the fish in the middle of the pan for about a few minutes each side or until it starts to change colour. Add the can of coconut milk or cream, whole cloves of garlic, coriander and simmer with the lid on for about 7-10 minutes in an oven on 160°C fan forced or 180°C electric. Best served in the pan.

BRAZILIANSTYLEFISH

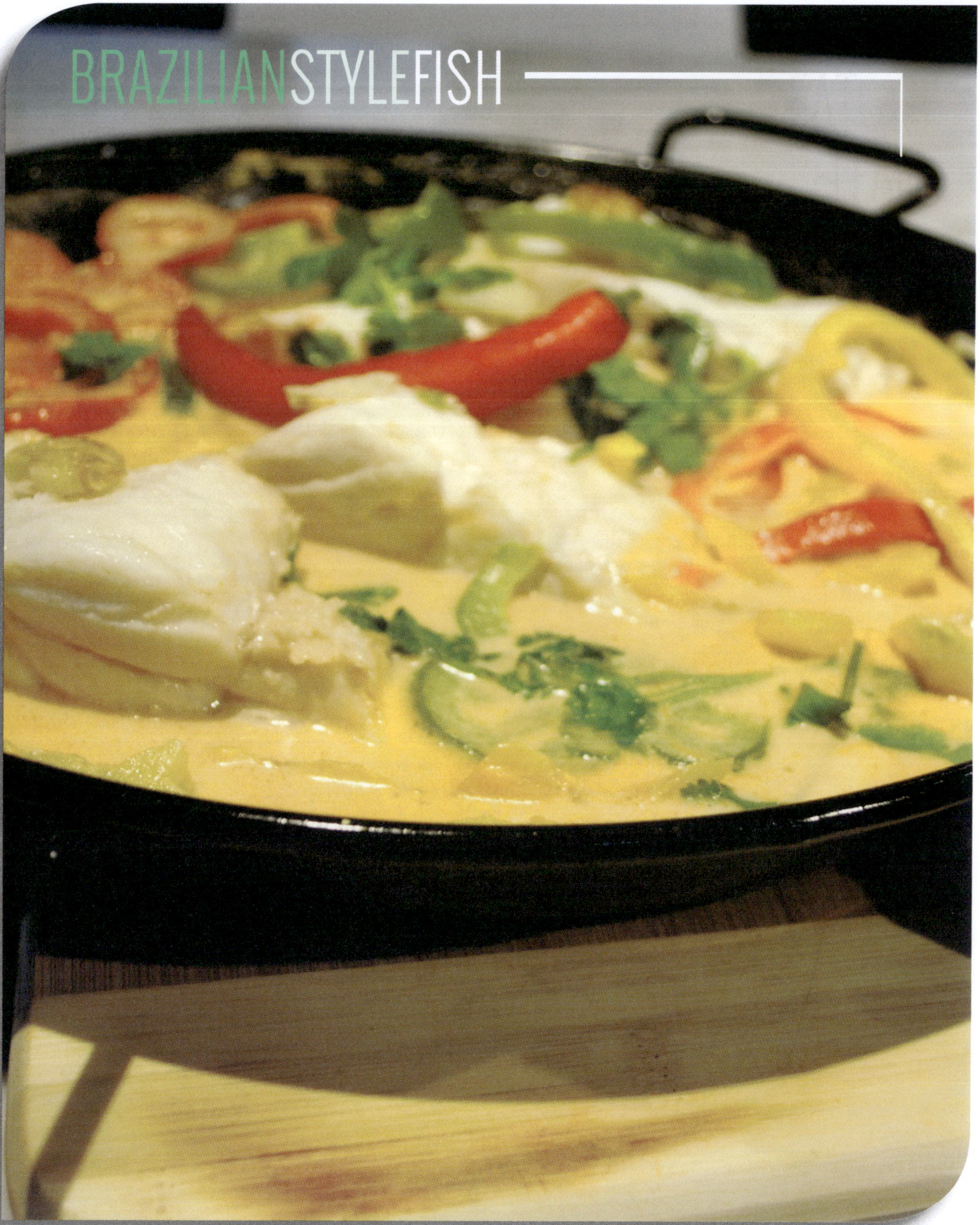

SILVERBEETANDCHICKENMASH-UP

Silverbeet and chicken mash-up served with Paleo protein pancakes

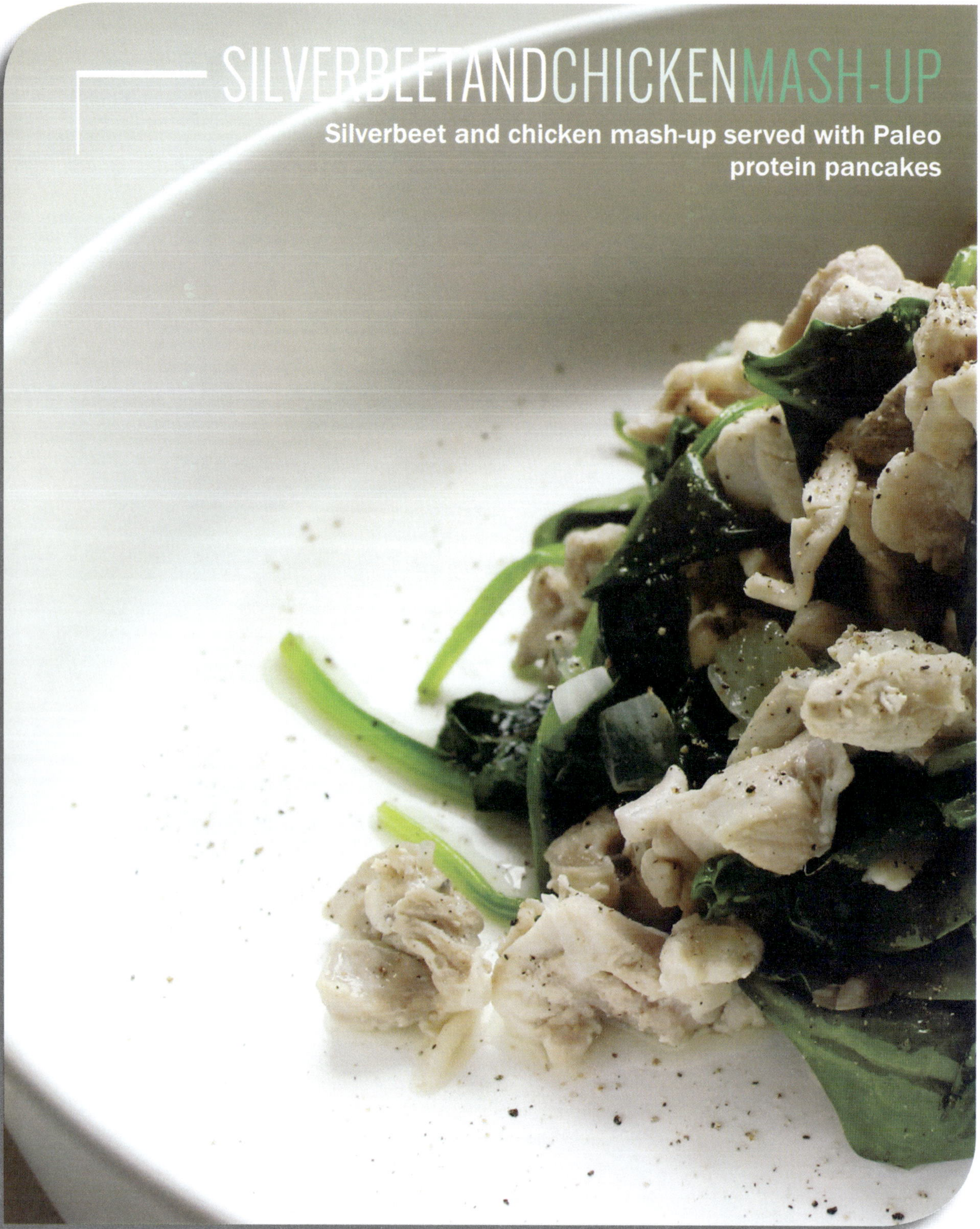

SILVERBEETANDCHICKEN MASH-UP

Serves 2

Ingredients

2 cups of cooked silverbeet, well chopped with liquid removed
1 onion finely diced
Protein of your choice - beans or chicken
2 tbls spelt flour
Pinch of salt and pepper
1/4 cup of water

MEXICANSTYLEOMELETTE

Serves 2

Ingredients

4 eggs
1/3 cup of milk
¾ cup of grated cheese (Tasty cheese is good)
½ red capsicum, chopped
2 spring onions, chopped
¼ cup parsley, chopped
Coconut butter to fry
Salt and pepper to season

Method

Whisk egg. Add milk, cheese, salt and pepper and mix well.

Heat coconut butter in a medium-sized fry pan. Pour in egg mixture and allow to cook for two minutes. Sprinkle over capsicum, onion and parsley and allow to cook for a further minute.

Roll up omelette ready to serve. Garnish with left over parsley.

**Note. You really can use any filling you desire. Avocado works equally well.*

MEXICAN STYLE OMELETTE

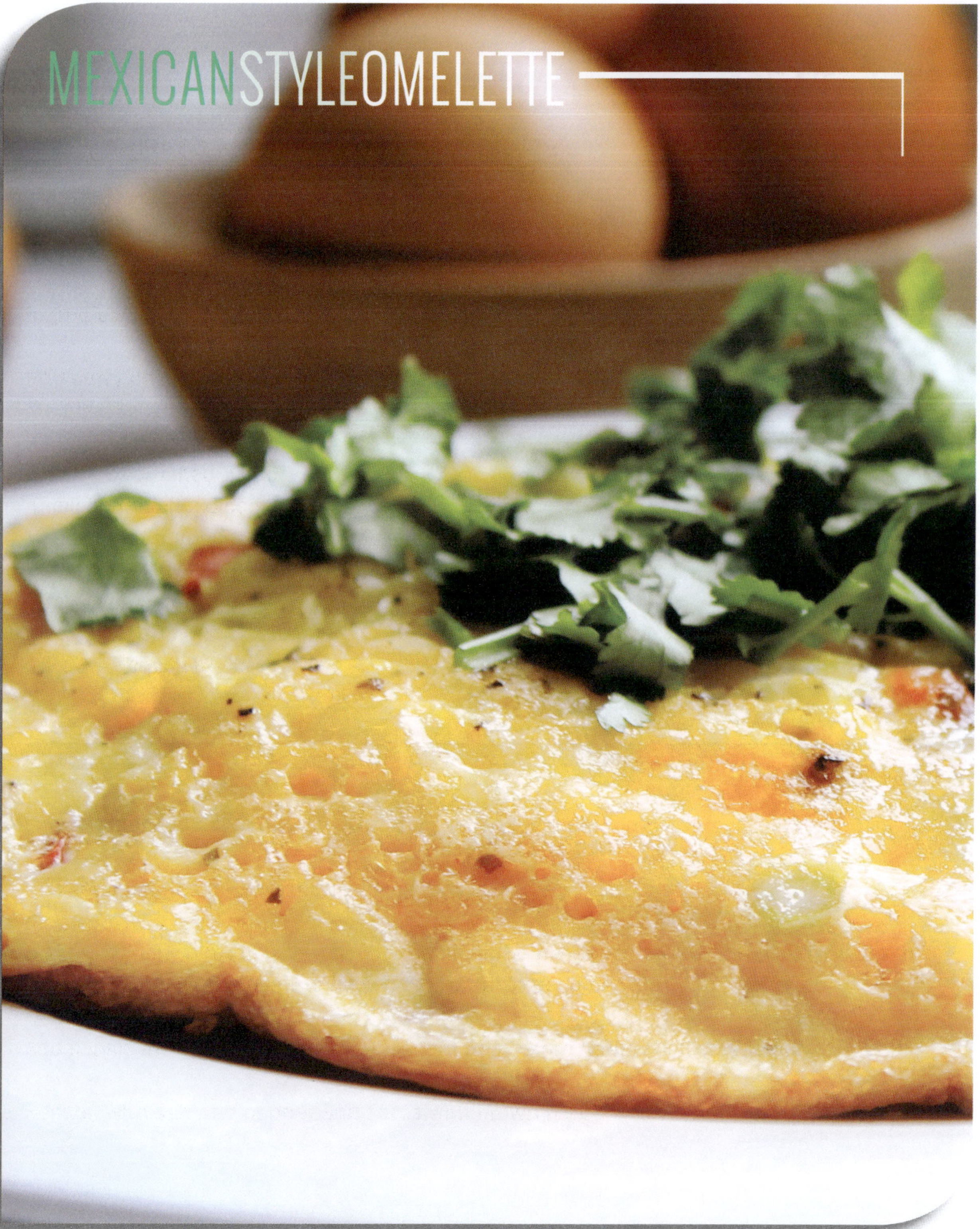

CHICKENANDPUMPKINCURRY

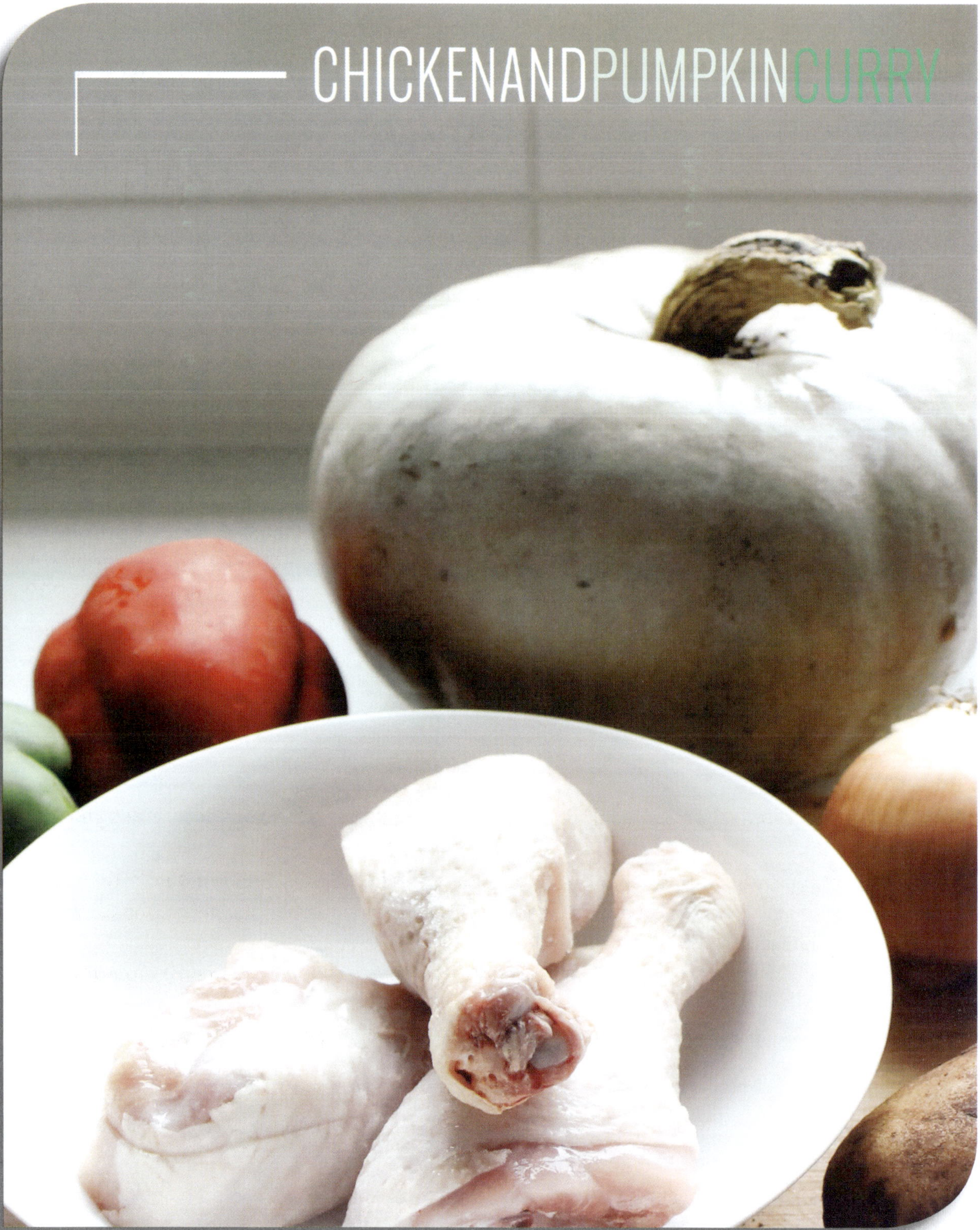

CHICKENANDPUMPKINCURRY

Serves 4

Ingredients

Red curry paste (it should just be herbs and spices with no sugar or anything else added – read the label)
1 onion, diced
1 piece of crushed garlic
4 chicken thighs, diced
½ butternut pumpkin, diced into 2cm cubes
2 potatoes, diced
1 red capsicum
1 bunch of spinach or similar
1 can of coconut milk
4 dates, chopped

Method

Use 2 tablespoons of curry paste and fry with oil in a pan until fragrant.

Add garlic and onion and stir.

Add pumpkin & potato, dates, coconut milk and if necessary a small amount of water to create enough liquid. Allow to cook until pumpkin becomes soft.

Add capsicum & cook for a further 3-4 minutes before adding fish and spinach.

Season with salt and pepper and serve with brown rice.

WINTERYSTEW

Serves 6

Ingredients

1 kg chuck steak
2 tbls coconut oil
1 onion roughly chopped
200 g mushrooms
1 sweet potato, peeled and chopped
3 cups stock
Parsley to serve

Method

In a large pot (preferably also ovenproof), add coconut oil and allow to melt.

Brown off steak and then add onion and mushroom and cook off until soft. Add sweet potato, 3 cups of stock and seasoning and then bring to the boil.

Move the pot to a moderate oven, allow to cook for 1 hour.

Serve with greens and garnish with parsley.

WINTERY STEW

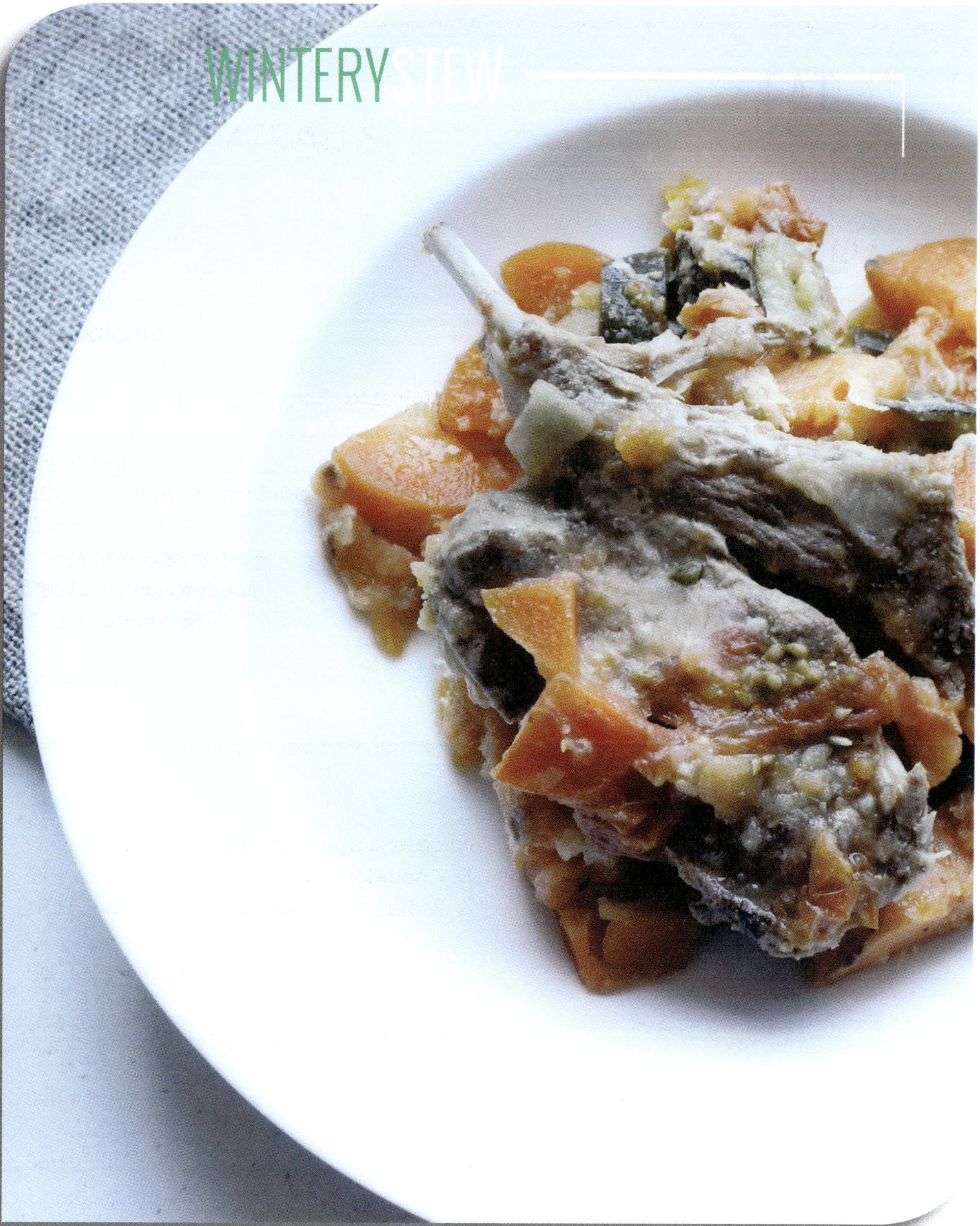

MIGHTY MEATBALLS

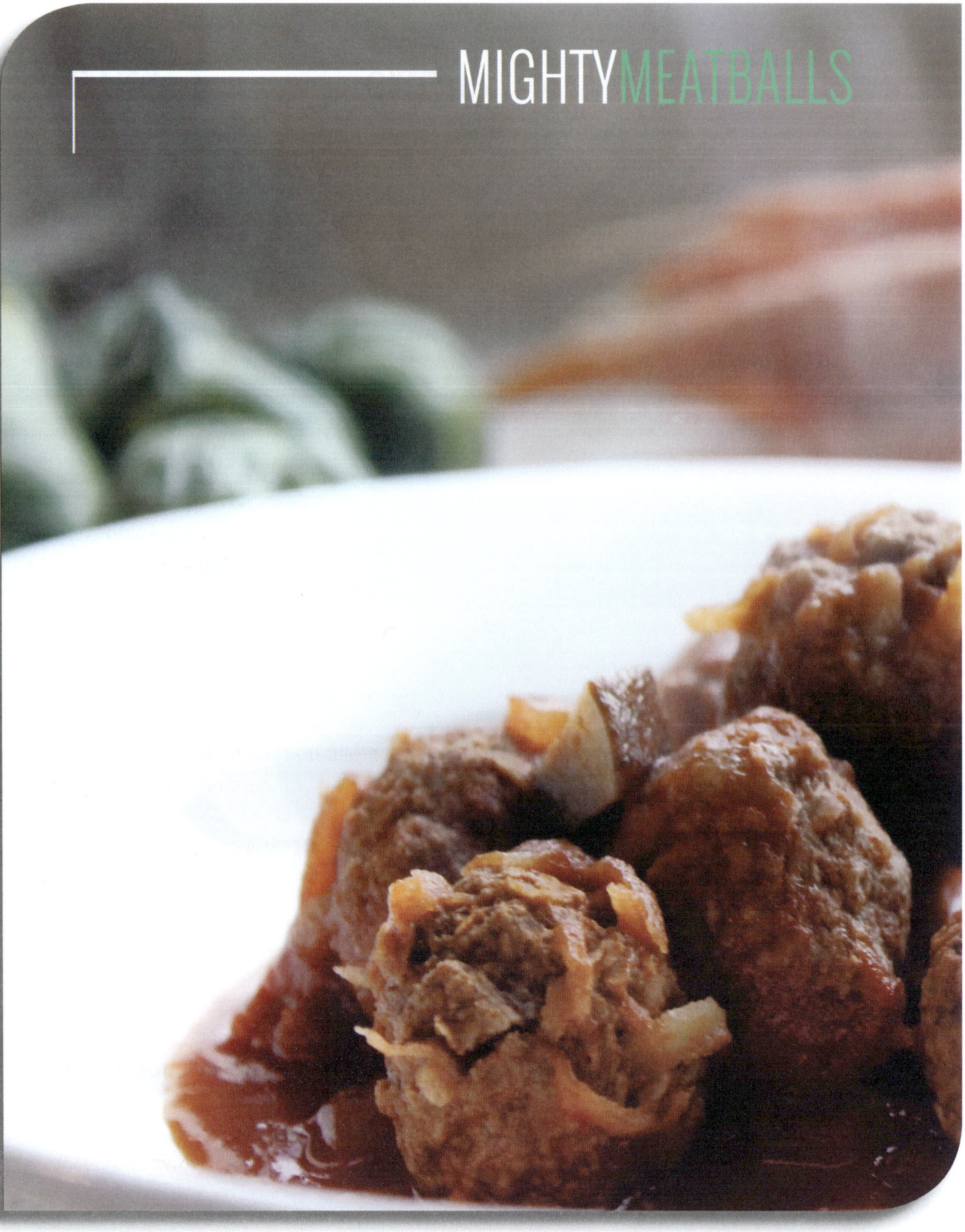

MIGHTYMEATBALLS

Serves 4

Ingredients

1 bottle of passata (preferably organic)
1 onion, diced
3 sprigs of basil
500 g of premium beef mince
2 eggs
50 g Parmesan cheese
Parsley finely chopped
2 tbls coconut oil

Method

Place coconut oil in a large saucepan. Add onion and fry until clear. Add passata and bring to a simmer.

Meanwhile, combine mince, eggs cheese and parsley and mix well with hands. Fill a bowl of water to submerse hands in between, rolling each meatball to prevent sticking and provide a wet layer around each meatball.

Roll mince mixture into meatballs.

Add meatballs gently to the passata mixture.

Simmer for 45 minutes.

Serve and garnish with basil.

CITRUSSALMON

Serves 4

Ingredients

2 salmon fillets of your choice
Juice of one lemon
1 small bunch of dill
Coconut oil
Salt & pepper to season

Method

In a baking tray, place salmon fillets side by side. Drizzle oil and lemon over fillets and arrange dill over the top.

Place in a moderate oven (180 °C) for 20 minutes or until just cooked. Serve with a side of greens.

Terms

tsp = teaspoon   tbls = tablespoon   SR flour = self-raising flour
g = grams

©All recipes copyright Andi Lew and Natalie Kringoudis

CITRUS SALMON

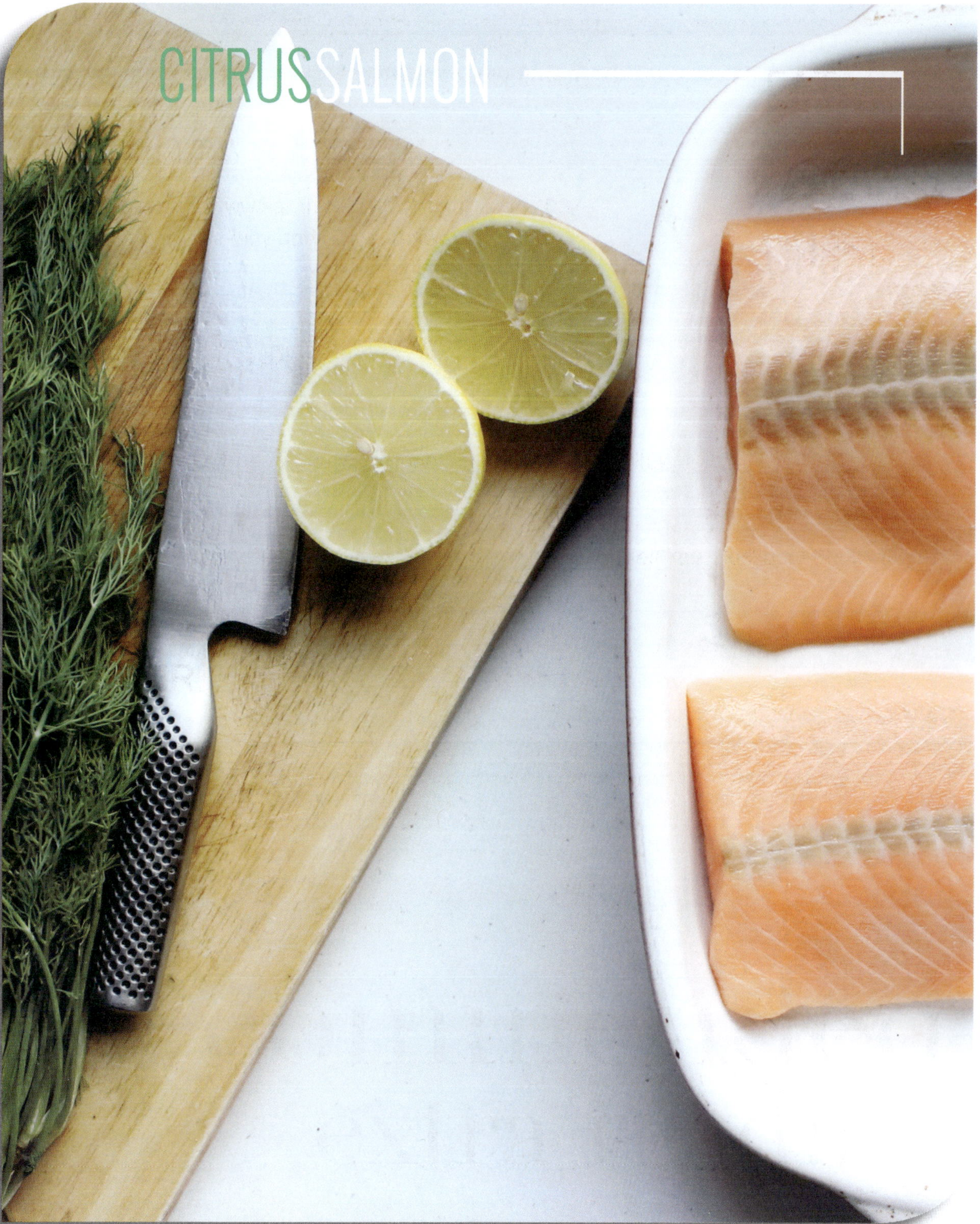

references &

CHAPTERONE

Cordian, L. (2002) *The Paleo Diet*. Hoboken, New Jersey. Wiley.

Fife, B and Kabara, Jon J. *The Coconut Oil Miracle*. Avery Trade

CHAPTERTWO

Gedgaudas, N. (2009) *Primal Body, Primal Mind*. 2nd Edition. Rochester, Vermont. Healing Arts Press.

Gullespie, D. (2010) *The Sweet Poison Quit Plan*. Melbourne, Australia. Penguin.

CHAPTERTHREE

Cordian, L. (2002). *The Paleo Diet*. Hoboken, New Jersey. Wiley.

Gullespie, D. (2010). *Sweet Poison*. Penguin.

Kringoudis, N. (2012). *Fertilise Yourself*. Melbourne, Australia. ini-inspire.

Wilson, S. http://www.sarahwilson.com.au/2011/03/caveman-exercise-a-why-and-how-rundown/

CHAPTERFOUR

Cordian, L. (2002). *The Paleo Diet*. Hoboken, New Jersey. Wiley.

Sipser, W & Lew, A. (2008). *7 Things Your Doctor Forgot to Tell You*. Rockpool Publishing

CHAPTERFIVE

Orr. A. (2007). *Concept Shen Seminar Notes*. Melbourne, Australia. Shen Therapies.

Wilson, S (2012). *I Quit Sugar*.

recommended extra reading

We are proud to announce our official Eat Fat Be Lean sponsor; Power Super Foods for all our salt, chia seeds and cacao as well as other complete super-foods, we recommend you too use them in our recipes.

They're not only a wonderful company, but they make quality products. Don't just take our word for it! Here's their promise to you:

Power Super Foods

Certified Organic · *Low G.I.* · *Fairly Traded* · *Vegan* · *Paleo* · *Raw* · *Gluten Free* · *Delicious*

www.powersuperfoods.com

Since 2001, Power Super Foods is Australia's premier source for the finest organic products specialising in organic, vegan, raw, Low GI, fairly traded, paleo, gluten-and-dairy-free functional foods.....our drive to lead the industry in introducing these unique foods to the Australian marketplace is appreciated by health conscious consumers around the country. We have traveled the globe (30+ countries !!) absorbing the ancient wisdom and searching for unique, traditional plants that provide energy and enhance wellbeing; we invite you to experience something new and enjoy adding these healthy traditions to your modern lifestyle, and will continue to introduce more and more intriguing functional foods and products as they come to our attention.

Our premium quality "superfoods" are always free of artificial preservatives or colours, and free of synthetic flavourings or additives helping you to meet your nutritional needs deliciously, naturally, and simply. We source our premium products through partnerships with farming communities around the world and pay a fair price to create economic opportunities among indigenous people in developing countries, supporting native agricultural traditions and helping to expand the development of good organic farming practices globally. Certified organic means they are grown without the application of petrochemical fertilisers or chemical pesticides, and are non-GMO and non-irradiated....the absence of all these elements speaks to the purity of the products.

This 100% Australian-owned company is committed to socially and environmentally responsible business practices, including hybrid company cars and carbon offsets every year. Part profits are donated annually to amazing organisations around the world devoted to changing this planet for the better in important arenas like endangered wildlife rehabilitation, empowering disadvantaged women, Tibetan causes, rainforest replanting, green energy & transport, etc. Power Super Foods is very proud to be a green, sustainable, progressive and planet-friendly business.

gourmetperuvianpinksalt

Peruvian Pink Salt has been hand harvested for over 2000 years from a natural ancient ocean spring bubbling up to the surface in theSacred Valley of the Incas near Machu Picchu, Peru at around 4000 metres above sea level. Pure salt sources are scarce today due to pollution of land and sea – ours is a low carbon footprint, evaporated product (not mined) and is carefully tested against heavy metal contamination.

This is the perfect healthy seasoning with a prized robust flavour and the rich mineralization creates a lovely pale pink colour, containing so many trace minerals including calcium, iron, potassium, magnesium, copper and zinc. The terraced salt ponds are owned by over 380 individual indigenous families, so why not enjoy gourmet quality flavour while assisting traditional local communities?

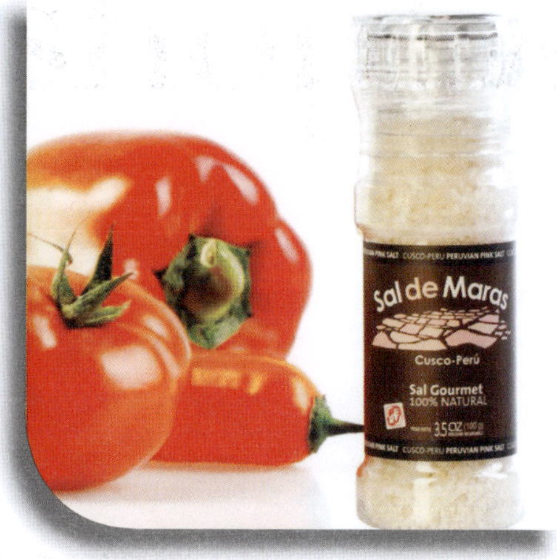

Serving suggestion: *Ideal for both gourmet cooking and everyday nutritional food preparation...great on just about everything! Check out our website for delicious healthy recipes where gourmet salt is a featured ingredient.*

SHOPPING DIRECTORY

you may be a little lost at first with where to shop and find these new pantry items. We want to make it easy to incorporate this healthy way of eating into your lifestyle.

At your local shopping centre most supermarkets now have an organic and health food section or aisle. You can find your organic produce there. Sugar alternatives are found in the sugar sections too with xylitol and stevia blends available right there at the supermarket. Your wheat-free baking flours may be in the health food section, and when choosing eggs, try to look for organic, not just free range, so you can be sure the chickens have been fed a natural diet free of hormones, pesticides or antibiotics. A great egg-free alternative for vegans is soaked chia seeds. Log onto www.powersuperfoods.com.au for the best chia seeds ever. When it comes to meat, try to buy hormone free and organic where possible.

You may also go to your local markets for organic produce, and more and more little health stores are popping up that will stock your organic cold-pressed coconut oils, wheat-free forage cereals to use for baking, as well as breakfasts, sugar free alternatives, wheat free flours and dairy alternatives.

FORAGECEREAL
PO Box 466 Hawthorn Victoria 3122
Australia
T. +61 03 9018 6639
www.foragecereal.com

THEPAGODATREE
2/124 Bridport Street Albert Park VIC
3206
T. (03) 9686 7454
www.thepagodatree.com.au

LOVINGEARTH
www.lovingearth.net

SIPSERFAMILYCHIROPRACTIC WELLNESSCENTRE
20 Ormond Rd Elwood VIC 3184
T. (03) 95313131
www.chiro4life.com

POWERSUPERFOODS
www.powersuperfoods.com.au

shape*up* & shop*here*

SHOPPINGDIRECTORY

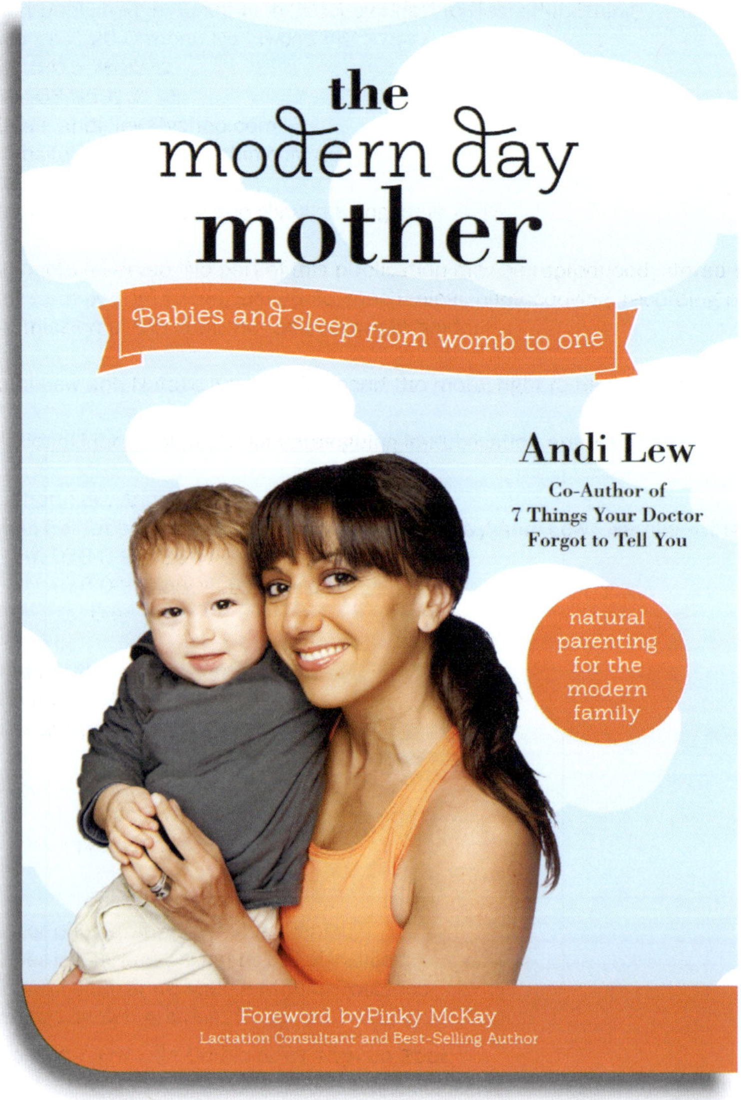

A guide to natural parenting for the modern family

- Easier pregnancy and birth
- Losing post baby weight
- Sleep solutions without tears
- Paediatric chiropractic
- Infant massage & bonding
- Understanding breastfeeding

"Strong evidence-based, it's beautifully supportive."

Pinky McKay, Lactation Consultant, best-selling author

"Such a gentle, lovely way of giving advice. It's the charm of the book."

Suzanne Male, journalist & author

"Andi presents Attachment Parenting in an easy-to-understand way."

Dr Bill Sears, best-selling author

Buy in e-book and paperback at www.themoderndaymother.com.

Also available for the Kindle at Amazon.com and from the Apple iBookstore

By Andi Lew

THEMODERNDAYMOTHER

FERTILISE YOURSELF

By Natalie Kringoudis

A book all about priming your body for fertility, featuring plenty of tips and tricks for a wellness overhaul and the 'how-to' steps to set yourself up to win.
If you're struggling with your fertility or even just your general health, this book can help you navigate your way to being fighting fertility fit!

With 25 recipes to help you build your fertile body this read will have your reproductive organs well on the road to babies in no time.

Foreword by Sarah Wilson.

"Nat has done a brilliant job at educating us on natural ways we can look at our fertility and overall health and wellbeing. This has been by far my favourite book on this important subject."

Melissa Ambrosini, Path to Wellness

http://melbournenaturalfertility.com.au/fertilise-yourself/

Also available from the Apple iBookstore and amazon.

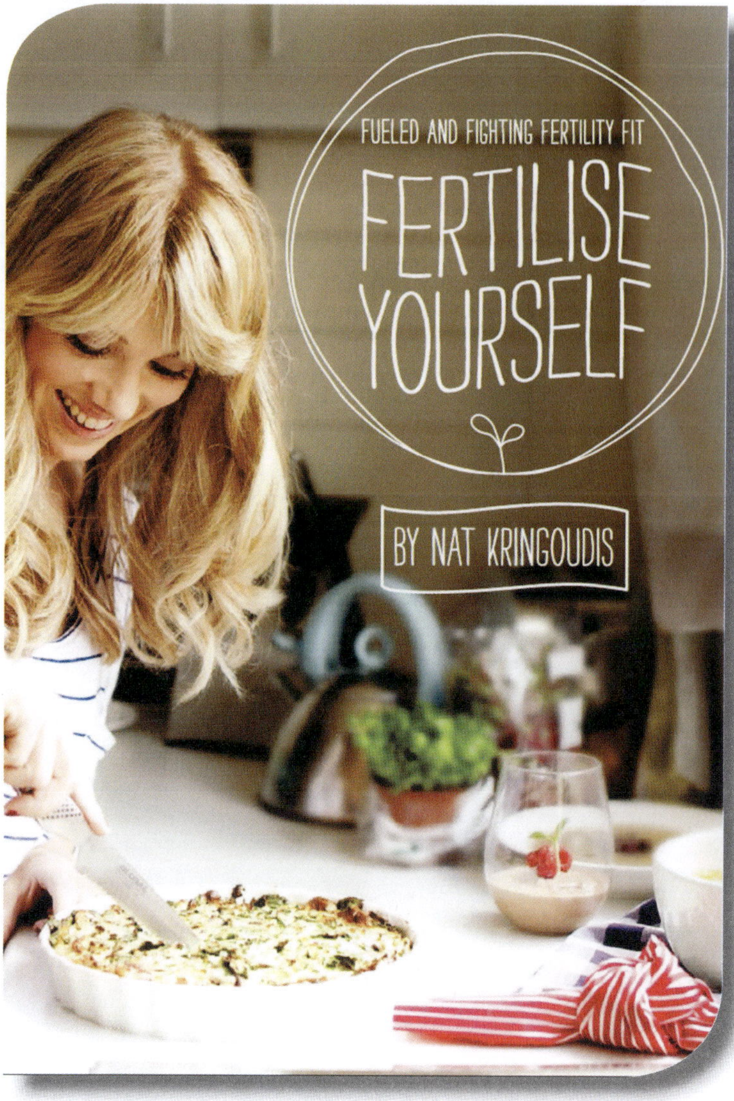

FAT&PROTEIN

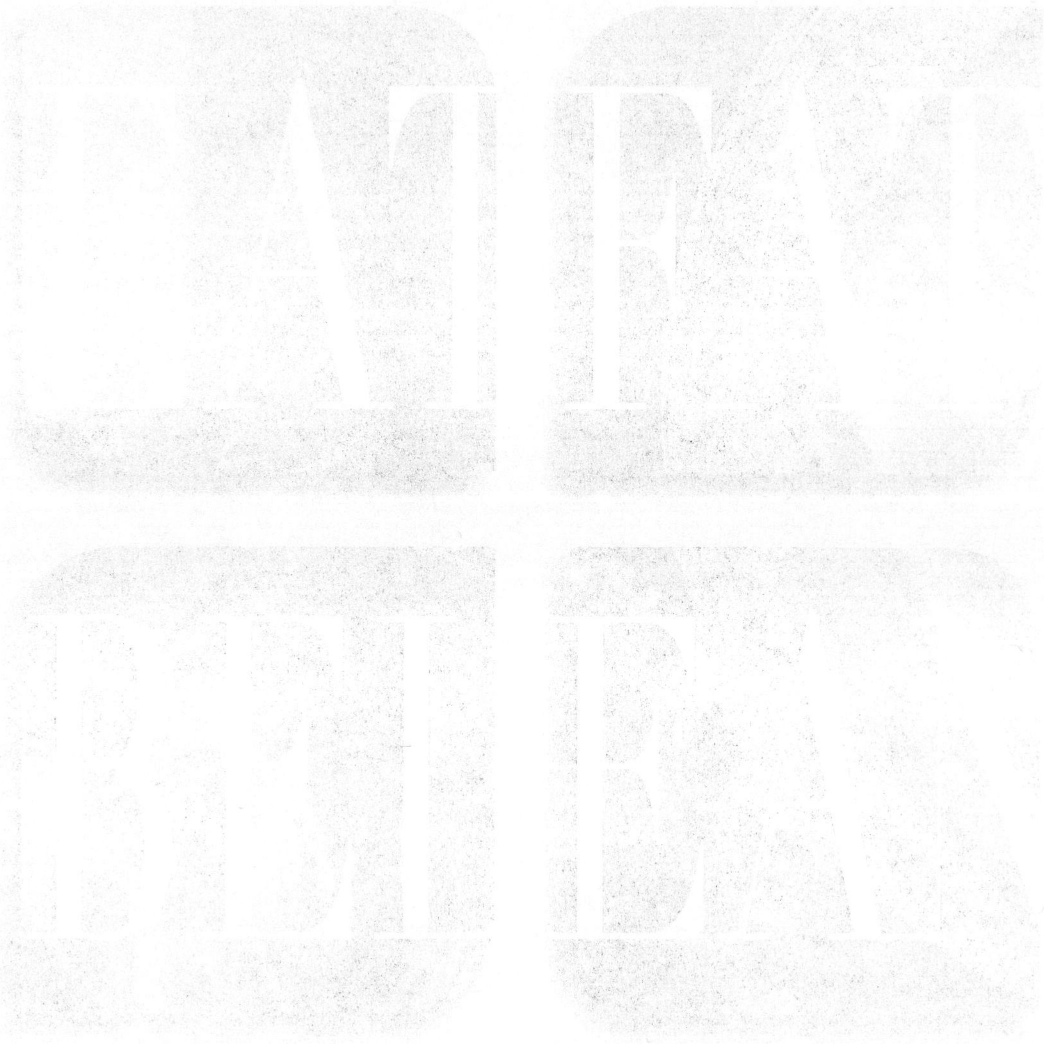

Printed in Dunstable, United Kingdom

91226143R00089